How to Stay Out of The Hospital

Excluding the need for medical emergency care, a routine trip to the hospital may either help or hinder the outcome. *How To Stay Out Of The Hospital* by Dr. Edward Wagner equips the reader with knowledge helpful in the decision-making process, with regard to conventional hospital care and an alternative approach. This book is a "must-read"; an "eye-opener"! I recommend it highly!

—*Dr. Paul G. Bogosian, B.A., D.C., Chiropractor*

How to Stay Out of The Hospital

The Kill or Cure Approach
The Only Business Successful Through Failure

Dr. Edward M. Wagner
with
Sylvia Goldfarb

Instant Improvement, Inc.
New York

The intent of this book is solely informational and is in no way meant to be taken as nutritional or medical prescription. Please consult a health professional should the need for one be indicated.

We occasionally mention a brand name product that has proven effective. We have no financial interest in these companies, nor do we receive any remuneration from them.

Instant Improvement, Inc.
210 East 86th Street
New York, New York 10028

Printed in the United States of America

Library of Congress Cataloging-in-Publication Data

Wagner, Edward M.
How to stay out of the hospital : the kill or cure approach : the only business successful through failure / Edward M. Wagner with Sylvia Goldfarb.
p. cm.
Includes index.
ISBN 0-941683-28-1
1. Medicine, Popular. 2. Alternative medicine. I. Goldfarb, Sylvia. II. Title.
RA82.W34 1996
610--dc20 96-16822

Dedication

To Barbara and Cookie
and all others like them,
who take responsibility for their own health
and search for the truth.

CONTENTS

Preface

How To Stay Out of the Hospital is a book of facts everyone should be aware of in order to take responsibility for their own health and be able to talk intelligently to their health care provider. It is a manual of alternative health facts. Our first book, *How To Stay Out Of The Doctor's Office, An Encyclopedia For Alternative Healing* is a treatment book.

The educational aspects of this book will give patients enough knowledge to be able to decide on a rational approach to treating their ailments in a viable non-threatening manner. The information is controversial and may likely cause negative feedback from the medical establishment which still insists upon magnifying ailments that are in most cases self-limiting. Stimulating a body's natural devices will help it to heal itself. By removing the cause of an illness, rather than using extreme methods to repair the damage, most people will be able to stay out of the hospital.

Patients will be able to decipher information that formerly would baffle and befuddle them and in many cases cause them to make a serious error in judgement. Of course, in cases such as accidents and acute medical emergencies, hospitals do an excellent job. In fact, emergency rooms in the United States are rated number one in the world.

However, for the treatment of chronic and degenerative ailments such as heart disease, diabetes, arthritis, depression, etc., not only does failure run rampant, but serious mistakes occur which in most cases are blatantly suppressed. Recent cataclysmic errors have caused death, disfigurement and suffering in an area that was supposed to provide healing and revitalization. Some alarming examples of when your own hospital becomes *your worst nightmare* follow.

In New York, a 50-year-old woman had a modified radical mastectomy after being mistakenly diagnosed with cancer. She became suspicious when the hospital refused to give her records to another doctor whom she had consulted about the possibility of postoperative chemotherapy. The error was made by the pathologists after a biopsy. When she sought a second opinion before undergoing the surgery, the consulting physician based his recommendation that she go ahead and have the surgery on the incorrect pathology report. Following the operation, the surgeon assured her that he got it all and that she should be thankful it was caught in the early stages.

After she learned she did not have cancer, she screamed, "You mean I didn't need the mastectomy? You mutilated my body for nothing!" The surgeon then remarked, "I haven't done anything wrong. I think I rendered the best treatment to that patient based on the facts which I had in my hand."[1]

In Michigan a mastectomy patient who did have cancer had the wrong breast removed.

A prominent medical writer in Boston with breast cancer was given a huge overdose of chemotherapy to the point that she regurgitated her own stomach lining and eventually died a hideous death. Another women was overdosed on chemotherapy in the same hospital and became permanently disabled.

It wasn't until a Texas man switched health plans and reviewed his medical records that he discovered his wrong lung had been removed at Osteopathic Medical Center of Texas.

The widow of a prominent composer was scheduled for hip replacement surgery. Due to a computer error a nurse asked her which knee it was. When the patient insisted it was her hip, not the knee, the nurse would not change the order without the doctor's permission. The doctor had to personally change it. He wrote the word "no" on each knee with a magic marker and the word "yes" on her right hip. This was a close call.

Another patient, in Florida, whose case was widely publicized, was not so lucky. His left leg was amputated below the

---

1.These quotes are from a tape of a program aired on radio station KYW in the Philadelphia area on November 2, 1995.

knee instead of his right leg which had severe circulatory problems. A malpractice lawyer said amputating the wrong limb is relatively rare since amputations are an uncommon procedure. But he says he has frequently sued due to cataract surgery being performed on the wrong eye or due to surgeons operating on the wrong part of a body.

This same surgeon, who took off the wrong leg, also amputated a patient's toe when she had agreed only to having dead tissue removed from her foot. He later denied doing so, stating that the toe had fallen off.

A New York woman died when her dialysis catheter was mistaken for a feeding tube and the doctor ordered food to be pumped into her abdomen.

After looking at a different patient's X-rays, the chief neurosurgeon at Memorial Sloan-Kettering Center in New York operated on the wrong side of a patient's brain.

And it isn't just surgeons who make mistakes. In a Maryland hospital, morphine instead of heparin (blood thinner) was administered to three infants. Incredibly they survived.

In a recent series investigating blunders and corruption in our medical system, *The New York Times* reported that, during a dialysis treatment, a patient named Sue screamed, pulled at her hair and vomited. Six hours later, she was dead, the tragic result of human error, and just one example of when hospitals kill.

A technician in the New Mexico hospital that was treating her had mistakenly thrown a switch to rinse the dialysis machine, not realizing Sue was still hooked up to it. The *rinse,* rather than the correct blood-cleansing solution, shot into her bloodstream, causing her cells to break apart.

But the nightmare didn't end there. Further investigation revealed that the dialysis machine was old and out-dated—without the security of the newer machines' alarm-warning system that would have saved her life.

The fact is, *The Times* investigation showed that, across the country, hospital equipment was either obsolete or inadequate, mostly for cost-cutting reasons. And this was in the face of questionable kickbacks and perks that made the income of doctors skyrocket.

Human error meets professional greed. The truth is, an American dialysis patient is *twice as likely to die* as a similar patient in Western Europe or Japan. Meanwhile our doctors are among the richest in the world.

The term "medical science" has become a contradiction in terms. Conventional medical care is often based on very little scientific proof, and it has been estimated that no more than 15 percent of medical and surgical intervention is supported by reliable scientific evidence.

A Harvard study published in 1991 concluded that nearly one of every 25 patients in New York State hospitals were injured by doctors or staff. In 1990 a study suggested doctors caused three times as many deaths in America as those killed by gunshots. And every year in America nearly 12,000 patients die from unnecessary surgeries. The numbers could very likely be even higher since malpractice lawyers often make settlement agreements that prevent injured patients from talking about their cases.

Unfortunately, physicians are trained and paid to treat illness rather than prescribe preventive measures. We are not saying that all medical and surgical procedures are unnecessary, but if we can enlighten the public as to what is mysteriously going on behind closed doors, they will be better able to make an informed and intelligent decision.

Knowledge is power. The information in this book will increase your knowledge, help allay your fears and prevent you from being exploited and intimidated into accepting arcane procedures, unnecessary, often dangerous, hospitalization and poisonous drugs that destroy your body's ability to recuperate naturally.

If you want a revolutionary alternative to the hazards of the hospital, read the health secrets and vital solutions in this book. The new generation of natural healers we talk about use natural methods so powerful, they can replace drugs, surgery and even hospitals. Let us show you how to take control of your own health now.

Should an occasion arise, however, when hospitalization is unavoidable, you will have a better chance of surviving your stay if you are well-informed. The conclusion of this book gives information that will enable you to protect yourself from the mishaps and inadequacies that often accompany hospitalization.

Acknowledgements

Our heartfelt thanks to our publisher, Eugene Schwartz, who believed in us and was willing to look at our proposal for our first book, *How To Stay Out Of The Doctor's Office,* which we sent in "over the transom." His encouragement, support and suggestions for both books were invaluable.

We would also like to add a special word of gratitude to our editor, Roberta Waddell, whose comments and queries about points that needed clarification helped to make this an even better book.

Introduction

The time has come for the public to realize that orthodox medical treatment is not working. Patients are considered conditions rather than human beings, and prolonging an illness has become more important than eventually curing it. High cost technology has changed the way medicine is practiced. The average time a doctor spends with a patient is five and a half minutes, barely enough time to say hello and good-bye.

Instead of healing the body, mind and spirit, patients are looked at piecemeal by specialists who know more and more about less and less. In contrast, a homeopathic practitioner spends three hours with a patient, taking an essential history. The reason for this is to learn about the person's constitution and determine how to best help the body rise above the illness.

In Europe 39 percent of all doctors use homeopathic methods and 60 percent of the people use homeopathic preparations. Many treatments proven successful in Europe have not been allowed into the United States. Pharmaceutical companies are instrumental in keeping these treatments from the American public because they are simple and inexpensive and would lessen their profits. Ironically, their stockholders are often the very people who are contracting illnesses and are in dire need of better treatment. Materialism in America has compromised integrity and betrayed the faith and hope of the people.

Before the age of super specialization, doctors cared more for their patients' welfare than for financial rewards. Physicians who deviate from the established methods are persecuted, have their licenses revoked and some have even been jailed. The public has lost freedom of choice in deciding what type of medical treatment they desire. Custody cases have been decided in favor of a parent who opts for conventional medicine. Case in point — Brian Ritchie, a rock star was awarded full custody of his son when a Milwaukee court ruled that the the child's mother endangered his health by choosing herbal treatments instead of steroids and antibiotics to treat his cystic fibrosis.

Pharmaceutical companies, the FDA and health insurance companies have placed such limitations on medical practitioners as to cause them to become less than adequate. Doctors forced into managed care programs cannot practice good medicine. With the advent of DRG's (Diagnostic Related Groups) patients are often booted out of hospitals before they are well enough to be cared for at home. For instance, instead of paying the hospital on a daily basis, the insurance companies allow the hospitals a flat rate for a particular surgical procedure, making it more profitable for the hospital to get the patient out quickly.

Chemotherapy is frequently used for certain cancers where statistics show it does not work. In many cases patients who have undergone chemotherapy and radiation refuse further treatment when the cancer returns because of the havoc brought upon their lives by this Middle Ages, inquisitional-type torture. Proven holistic methods are not allowed since they cannot be patented and therefore are not profitable.

"Watchful waiting" is a term that often contributes to the ongoing process of an illness. The definition of watchful waiting is that a serious condition has been diagnosed and that nothing should be done to alleviate it at the present time. Women are often told a small breast tumor appears to be non-threatening. Biologically, cancer is an insidious disease that eventually grows out of control and, if left to its own devices, will spread through the body and eventually destroy it. If, after a period of watchful waiting, it is determined that a malignancy is indeed present, horrendous devastating treatment modalities are instituted, causing undue suffering and devastating pain.

If this same woman had been seen by a holistic physician, a detoxifying process would have been instituted immediately. She would have been checked for heavy metals, investigated for deficiencies of vitamins, minerals and amino acids and would have her diet adjusted. A psychological investigation would be performed. An explanation would be given to her regarding changes that would have to be made in her attitude to eliminate the ongoing, relentless stress of facing the adversities of life. Through this method, the chance of her condition becoming a life-threatening one would be reduced by almost 90 percent.

Many patients with no symptoms are told that immediate treatment is needed for a condition that is not affecting their lives. Using fear tactics, doctors intimidate a healthy patient so much that the patient actually starts to think like a sick person, stimulating a course of disease that was originally only an illusion. Case in point: A 49-year-old civil engineer with severe headaches went to the hospital for a diagnosis and was told he had three blocked coronary arteries. He had been living a physically active life style with very little stress. Golf and tennis were regular activities. He was told not to leave the hospital, to contact his family and put his affairs in order. A triple bypass would be performed within days. Through fear and intimidation, he agreed to have the procedure and unfortunately became one of the five percent to succumb during the surgery—another example of when hospitals kill.

A great injustice to patients is to be told by a doctor that they have only a limited time to live. No person has the right to dictate to another how long they have to reside on this planet. Only God determines that. Most of the public has little or no knowledge how the body functions and can be easily intimidated into believing that whatever the doctor tells them is gospel. It becomes a self-fulfilling prophesy. Telling a person he or she has three months to live plants a seed in their mind that eventually destroys them. The doctor has committed a crime equal to murder, yet suffers no fear of prosecution from the legal authorities.

In contrast to orthodox physicians, holistic doctors do not engender high remuneration and have more of a personal interest in their patients who step into a world of renewed health and peace of mind. Far too many orthodox doctors, in their need for acceptance by the system, sell their souls at the cost of their integrity and thus betray the dignity of a once proud profession.

The medical system has made us a nation of worriers. It is pathetic that the American public constantly carries the fear of debilitation and death through terminal illness. We are accosted at every corner by the media encouraging us to seek treatment and medication for a myriad of conditions. Not a day goes by without hearing of the threat of terminal cancer, bypass surgery, amputation of limbs or diabetes. This constant harassment bombards our peace of mind enough to make us paranoid and psychologically inept. Life is stressful enough without these added threats to our health and well-being.

Fear and worry must be eliminated in order for a person's immune system to have the ability to fend off the viruses, bacteria and environmental factors encountered in every aspect of life. We are taught that sickness and ill health is bad. This is promulgated by the authorities for the continuation of positive economics, with no regard for the individual's well-being. Rather than clinging to the philosophy of life as good or evil or sick or well, we should adopt a neutral attitude. *Illness should be regarded as the body's effort to rid itself of toxins. Instead of inundating our bodies with poisonous drugs, symptoms should be thought of as a way of warning us that changes have to be made in our lifestyle.* Traumatic experiences ought to be regarded as teaching tools rather than times of tremendous despair and hopelessness.

People do not realize that, when they are ill, the cause could be other than a virus or bacteria. Throughout my experience of healing, I have recognized one main ingredient that stands out in an individual's personality. This ingredient is selfishness. Most people I see with illnesses, especially the more serious ones, are not happy people. I have yet to see a person who is truly happy and sick at the same time. Happiness and illness are incompatible due to the fact that happy people have a strong impetus to survive and utilize the potential they have to offer society.

In contrast, sick people are so involved with their illness that they disregard everything and everyone, including the loved ones who surround them. They talk about themselves with such passion as to think they are the only ones who live upon the earth. They only want to hear about themselves and are not interested in anyone else's problems. This attitude produces negative vibrations and does not allow these individuals the benefit of the positiveness that surrounds them. Other people shy away from them and do not accept them, causing extreme unhappiness leading to a downward cycle of ill health.

Orthodox treatment often causes more of a problem than the original disease. Patients with high blood pressure are frequently placed on blood-pressure-lowering medication without investigating the cause of the problem. With complete disregard for the biochemical activity of the body and a desire for a quick fix, the rote system is to write a prescription. In fact, if patients leave the doctor's office without a handful of prescriptions, they are disappointed.

What is not understood by the orthodoxy is that certain minerals are needed to activate enzymes directly responsible for the body's own production of blood-pressure-lowering chemicals. The diuretics prescribed flush these minerals out of the system which, in turn, causes an exacerbation of the original blood pressure problem. Essential enzymes become depleted and dysfunctional because of the toxicity of the patient's system. When the system is toxic, oxygen cannot nourish the enzymes, which then become deactivated.

Loss of oxygen also allows viruses, bacteria and pathogens to overproliferate since they depend on a low oxygen environment for their survival. With adequate oxygen present, the enzymes keep these invaders in check. If the true problem, the toxicity of the system, were addressed, there would be no need for medication since the body would then produce its own blood-pressure-regulating chemicals.

This proven scientific fact applies to every malfunction in the body. The holistic practitioner would initially incorporate a detoxifying program to clear the body of unnecessary toxins, thereby allowing the immune system to be strengthened, which allows the body to heal itself.

Why does our country allow a regulatory commission to use Gestapo-like tactics in the invasion of our freedom of privacy by raiding health food stores and holistic doctors' offices? Millions of people are dependent on nutritional supplements for longevity and the extension of the high quality of their lives. A case in point would be a 47-year-old regional sales manager who had undergone orthodox treatment for a heart problem. Besides doing nothing to alleviate the problem, the therapy affected his lifestyle to such a degree that it made him partially immobile and unable to work. When I first saw this formerly active individual, he had become lethargic and depressed. Through the use of natural supplements, however, he was able to overcome the disabilities which were caused by the medications and is now living a normal life.

However, the FDA, in their infinite wisdom, decided these supplements were drugs and removed them from the free market under the auspices of protecting the public. This has led to the eventual death or severe debilitation of countless similar patients. In essence, the FDA committed murder while protected by the political system. Our system allows pharmaceutical companies to employ lobbyists to fatten their pocketbooks with complete disregard for the health and welfare of the American public.

The lobby system in the United States is a blight on our so-called free competition, which allows for monopolies to stifle opposition. A hundred million Americans contacted their senators and representatives imploring them to pass two bills pertaining to availability of nutritional supplements and for freedom of choice in their selection of medical treatment.

These bills were stymied by the conflict of interest of two of the leading congressmen who, because of their own egotistical needs, decided that their opinion was more important than that of the public. But the bills passed anyway, thanks to the public *not* under the thumb of the lobbyists.

This book is an effort to decry the methods and manipulations of the select few intent upon controlling the masses. Through knowledge and consumer's groups like those that helped keep supplements available, the system can be returned to its original intent prescribed by our founding fathers.

Two hundred years from now the medical authorities will look back in dismay at the archaic procedures and medications that are now in use.

It is our fervent hope that this book will be a step forward in enlightening the public about the lies that have been foisted on them by an increasingly corrupt system.

Part I

- *FDA*
- *Fallacies And Misrepresentations Of Medical Gospel*
- *Orthodox Propaganda*

1 FDA — The Double Standard

Why does the FDA prevent companies manufacturing vitamins and supplements from making claims for their products but allow pharmaceutical companies to make claims for their products that sometimes are not true and have often killed people? This is a double standard that should not be allowed in a democratic system.

FDA Should Be Indicted For Murder

The FDA is more concerned with stopping alternative therapy than it is in the patients' welfare. A case in point is the use of Cancell, an alternative treatment for cancer that was used successfully in treating 10,000 patients. The FDA stopped distribution of Cancell by citing interstate commerce regulations. These did not really apply since Cancell was distributed at no charge. Since then, many people being kept alive by Cancell have died unnecessarily. If the function of the FDA is to protect the public, why is it destroying so many people?

Most Orthodox Treatments Never Proven

According to a 1978 study by the Office of Technological Assessment (OTA), *80 percent of orthodox therapy has never been authenticated by double blind studies.* Yet, the orthodoxy constantly denigrates complementary medicine and alternative healing modalities for not performing double blind studies. One reason this is not done is that only the pharmaceutical companies have enough money to sustain an ongoing study of any medication or treatment which can often cost over 100 million dollars and take 10 years.

Combining Drugs Dangerous

Drugs are tested singly and not in combination with each other, yet many patients are prescribed several drugs at a time. Combinations should be tested.

FDA's Tunnel Vision

Certain nutrients have to be smuggled into the United States from Europe. The idea that another culture has answers the failure-prone American doctors don't have is beyond the FDA's comprehension.

Alternative Medicine Reduces Health Costs

The German National Health System permits the use of alternative medicine. This has greatly reduced health care costs compared to the United States where the FDA does not allow alternative methods.

German Chemotherapy Zaps Tumor—Spares Healthy Tissue

Dr. Hans Neiper of Germany uses Interlipid, a substance that directs the chemotherapy directly to the tumor instead of inundating the entire body with massive amounts of a toxic substance. This lessens the horrendous side effects of chemotherapy.

Public Sabotaged

Migraine medication works on the principle of reproducing serotonin (a mood modulator in the brain). Serotonin is derived from the amino acid tryptophan which is derived from animal foods. Not only did the medical establishment frighten the public into limiting their intake of animal-type foods, they also pulled supplements of tryptophan from the shelves of the health food stores at about the same time that the new antidepressant medication PROZAC was being introduced.

Baby Food Contains Outlawed Supplement

Tryptophan was pulled out of the health food stores in 1990. It has never been allowed back in this country to be used as a supplement. Yet, it is present in baby food and formulas and it was not removed from the shelves in Canada.

Natural Blood Thinners

If aspirin were a new drug on the market, the FDA would ban it because of its harmful side effects (bleeding ulcers and blood-thinning properties). In place of aspirin, the following supplements can be used for blood thinning: Vitamin C, fish oil, garlic and bromelain. Take bromelain on an empty stomach.

Therapist Defies Gestapo

Jane Priestly, who operates an AIDS clinic in Los Angeles, has the best statistics in the country for the treatment of AIDS. She does not use AZT, DDI or any other medications. Priestly uses natural nutrients which will be taken off the market if the FDA is allowed to continue their Gestapo-like tactics in not allowing the American public to choose how they wish to be treated.

Scare Tactics

The FDA does not want nutritional supplements to take away the public's incentive to purchase drugs. In its love affair with the drug companies, the FDA uses a process of fear and intimidation to dissuade the American public from utilizing the positive effect of nutrients in place of medication that, in most cases, is ineffective and often debilitating.

Is The FDA Protecting Us?

Why doesn't the FDA protect us from the mercury in dental fillings, the alcohol in the bars and liquor stores, the cigarettes in the vending machines, the drugs on the street and the terrible side effects of chemotherapy and other injurious medications, instead of harassing us about vitamin supplements which have always been effective without side effects and which aid us in fending off such terrible diseases as cancer, multiple sclerosis, diabetes and lupus?

FDA Would Not Approve Aspirin Today

Suppose a new medication were introduced this year that was an effective pain reliever, reduced headaches and fever and helped ease joint pain. However, anyone taking this medication several times a day would have a high incidence of gastric or intestinal bleeding and thirty thousand people a year would suffer side effects severe enough to require hospitalization. Would the FDA approve this medication? Of course not. Yet it is available to both young and old alike with no restrictions. What we are describing is aspirin.

FDA Delays Effective Treatment

The FDA is notoriously slow in approving health claims. An example is the recently announced health claim for folic acid to prevent birth defects. The FDA had this information for the past ten years, but sat on it. It is unreasonable and unconscionable that this information was not given to women of childbearing age because folic acid supplementation could have prevented innumerable, irreversible birth defects in those ten years.

FDA Sides With Big Bucks

The FDA attempted to remove amino acids from the shelves of the health food stores and make them available only by prescription. Yet, NutraSweet contains two amino acids, aspartic acid and phenylalanine, in addition to methanol, a wood alcohol which causes seizures and convulsions. A quart of beverage sweetened with NutraSweet contains 250 mg of phenylalanine.

FDA Prefers Toxic Treatment

Basil Wainright, a British scientist living in Florida, has been in prison for years without a trial or conviction. His crime — the invention of an ozone machine that has been proven through peer review and scientific studies to cure cancer and AIDS. The FDA confiscated his work and equipment because they have complete disregard for natural healing methods. They are more concerned with the use of toxic drugs which, statistically, have been proven failures.

FDA Blind To Canadian Studies

Latest studies from the Manitoba Institute of Cell Biology in Canada show three allergy medications, Hismanal, Claritin and Atarax, showed an increase in cancer at low dosages in animal studies. Yet, the FDA refutes this information and says there is no cause for alarm.

DMSO Outlawed In Health Food Stores

DMSO is prescribed by physicians for the treatment of interstitial cystitis (a painful bladder condition), yet it cannot be purchased in health food stores as a topical treatment for arthritis and/or inflamed joints.

2 Fallacies And Misrepresentations Of Medical Gospel

Beware of the fallacies and misrepresentations promoted by orthodox medicine to keep from the public from the truth about ineffective testing, unnecessary surgery, overmedication and a multitude of inconsistencies that may cause undue pain and even death.

Ineffective Medications

Recent studies show no significant benefit using quinine for nocturnal leg cramps or antibiotics for bronchitis, yet they are still prescribed.

Sore Throat—The Often Unrecognized Cause

Frequent sore throat could be due to esophageal reflux. Stomach acids rise and irritate the throat. Patients are often misdiagnosed and unnecessarily treated with antibiotics, when 2 ounces of aloe vera gel taken 3 times a day is almost 100 percent effective.

Leftovers With Surgical Procedures

A woman was spitting up blood following a mastectomy. Years later a chest X-ray revealed that a clamp had been left in her body during the surgery. Many incisional abscesses are due to material left in the body during surgery. Patients with unusual post-surgical symptoms should demand their X-rays and review them with an impartial physician.

Some Sodium And Cholesterol Are Good For Your Health

The tendency of human nature is to go from one extreme to another. When people are told that too much of a substance is bad for their health, they often stop using it entirely. First, sodium was the culprit; then it was cholesterol, two substances the body needs in moderation to function properly.

Many older people suffer from heat exhaustion as a side effect of their blood pressure medication. This depletes the body of sodium, a mineral necessary to retain water and prevent dehydration.

People fear cholesterol as something dangerous when, in fact, it is needed for many important bodily functions. The membrane of the cells, especially brain cells, the myelin sheath which insulates nerve fibers, and the adrenal glands which produce 50 life-supporting steroids, are all made from cholesterol. It is also necessary for production of bile in the liver for digestion.

Also, menopausal side effects can be due to a lack of cholesterol which the body needs to manufacture estrogen in other organs after the ovaries have ceased functioning and producing it.

Long-Term Effects Of Medication

No one knows about the long-term effects of medications that are new on the market. Most are tested only from three to six months.

Doctors' Families Nix Chemotherapy

Why is it that some medical doctors send their family members to foreign countries for cancer treatment, rather than subject them to the horrendous side effects of chemotherapy and radiation? Instead of these, holistic therapy is used on their family members with excellent results. Yet, these same doctors still prescribe chemotherapy and radiation to their patients in the United States.

Frightening Medical Hype

People are so frightened by hype from the medical establishment that they panic at the least little symptom and immediately rush to the doctor. Chances are that a battery of tests will be ordered which, in most cases, are unnecessary. Many of these tests are invasive and can cause a problem that wasn't there in the first place. In addition they cause people to worry about the results which, in turn, depresses the immune system. And some doctors make frightening statements, causing undue worry that can depress the immune system and lead to illness. Most symptoms are self-limiting and will disappear in a short time if left alone. A healthy body has the ability to restore itself if left alone. Of course, in certain instances, such as chest pain or sudden loss of vision, people should seek medical help.

Pharmaceutical Companies Rob The Public

The same drug used for deworming animals was found to be effective in treating colon cancer in humans. It cost 6 cents per pill to treat animals. Even though there was no change in the formula and no additional cost to the pharmaceutical companies, the cost skyrocketed to $ 6.00 per pill when it was used to treat humans.

Epilepsy Cases Increase

Epilepsy has increased 500 percent since DPT shots were started in the 40s, not a coincidence.

Too Many Tetanus Shots

No more than three tetanus shots should be given during a lifetime because the accumulated effect of the tetanus virus that is injected eventually causes the body to store so much of the virus that it can actually increase susceptibility to the disease.

Nicotine Patches

Nicotine patches can cause insomnia and weird dreams.

Immune System Hexed By Diagnosis

When someone is told he or she has a disease, the diagnosis itself is more traumatic than the actual symptoms. The diagnosis causes a fear response leading to a depressed immune system accompanied by pain that is more related to stress than to the disease itself.

Prophylactic Use Of Antibiotics

People with mitral valve prolapse are routinely given antibiotics to protect the heart when they have dental work performed.

However, prostate examinations and vaginal examinations also cause mitral valve prolapse, but patients are not given antibiotics for these procedures.

Crimes Against The Elderly

Overmedication of the elderly is more of a problem than street drugs. What is diagnosed as Alzheimer's disease is often the side effect of medication.

Off-Key Blood Tests

Blood tests performed for electrolyte balance (potassium, sodium, magnesium and calcium) are only 50 percent accurate.

No Symptoms No Treatment

Patients who have no symptoms, but are told they must be treated for a disease, often suffer serious side effects from the treatment which could eventually lead to death. If these patients were to institute a nutritional health program and follow a healthy lifestyle, their disease would not progress. In fact, it could be completely reversed and their quality of life increased.

Double Standard Affects Holistic Practitioners

Fifty thousand people a year die of malnutrition in hospitals at the hands of dietitians and doctors, and not a word is said. But if one person were to die from an overdose of vitamin supplements (which has never happened), a furor would be raised that could destroy a practitioner's career and future.

Hi-Tech Replaces Personal Touch

Many doctors treat laboratory results rather than their patients.

Hospital's Convenience More Important Than Patient's Welfare

Use of the urinary catheter can lead to scarring and narrowing of the urethra and can cause bacterial infections at a later date. Catheters are more often used for the convenience of hospital personnel rather than for the patients' welfare.

Naturopathic Docs Score A Win

The United States has 2000 naturopathic (Natural Healing) physicians compared with 50,000 in Europe. Although naturopathic physicians have higher rates of success treating almost every condition, this disparity shows that, even though something is effective, it is not allowed in this country unless it is scientifically proven. In Germany, ozone therapy to destroy viruses in the body is paid for by insurance companies. Results have been excellent in the treatment of cancer and AIDS.

Double Blind Studies Unfair

Double blind studies are just a ploy to sell and verify pharmaceuticals because only the drug companies have enough money to perform these studies. In double blind studies, neither the doctor nor the patient knows who is getting the real medicine and who is getting the placebo. If you take part in a double blind study, would you want to be the one receiving the placebo? This type of study is immoral.

Overmedication Poisons The Elderly

Overmedication of the elderly can result in kidney disease if arteriosclerosis is present. The medicine concentrates in the kidneys and, if they are not functioning properly, the medicine will poison the system instead of just passing through it.

Antihistamines Poison Blood

Antihistamines slow the pace of urinary elimination and this can lead to blood toxicity.

Dangerous Shots

Only 60 people in the United States died from chicken pox in 1992. Yet, vaccinations are being recommended for the entire population of 260 million people. More complications can take place from the vaccinations than from the disease.

Beware Of Human Growth Hormone

Beware of using Human Growth Hormone for its anti-aging properties. The down side is that HGH is only one part of the anabolic cascade[1] and, without other compatible hormones, most of it is not properly utilized. When it is not, the HGH goes directly to the ends of the bones, the nose, jaw and ears, causing them to grow. It also builds a shelf of bone above the eyes and opens gaps between the teeth as the jaw grows.

Marijuana Should Be A Prescription Item

Marijuana is a potent antispasmodic and is useful in treating multiple sclerosis, spinal cord injuries, cerebral palsy, trigeminal neuralgia and herniated discs. It can give immediate relief from the nausea associated with chemotherapy. Since it is smoked, it is absorbed directly into the bloodstream, a plus for patients who are so nauseated they can't hold down oral medication.

Despite its effectiveness, the government has suppressed research on marijuana, forcing patients to obtain it by illegal means. Unlike narcotics, marijuana does not suppress the respiratory system. Certain people who use a great deal of marijuana have extremely low incidences of glaucoma. The side effect of marijuana is a feeling of exultation. Note: I am not advocating the indiscriminate use of marijuana for recreational purposes.

Say No To A Tonsillectomy

Inflammation of the tonsils is usually caused by a food allergy, most likely dairy (milk) products. After weaning or age three, children should not drink milk. The public has been misinformed that milk is necessary. Milk contains too much phosphorus, which actually stops calcium absorption. In addition, milk's fat content is too high for humans. In six months a calf's weight increases by a factor of eight.

Tonsils are an integral part of the immune system and without them the immune system is compromised. In addition, tonsil tags (tissue left following tonsillectomy) can harbor bacteria

---

1. There is both an anabolic and catabolic cascade. During the catabolic cascade, energy is being released from the cells due to a high acid condition. During the anabolic cascade, the cells are resting and in an alkaline state. This makes the human growth hormone more effective since it has less opposition.

which can cause infections and inflammation in other parts of the body.

"First Do No Harm"

At one time all doctors in the United States belonged to the AMA. Nowadays only 25 percent are members. The reason is that some physicians find the AMA to be too bureaucratic. In addition, many feel the organization's philosophy is compromising to the Hippocratic Oath (First do no harm). Many have turned to a more holistic approach which entails the treatment of the entire system, including body, mind and spirit.

Routine Procedures Unproven

Rigorous scientific studies show that only 10 to 20 percent of all routine medical and surgical procedures in the United States have been proven effective.

Cancer/Steroid Connection

Growth hormones and anabolic steroids will increase the growth of cancer in the body.

Don't Tinker With Your Nasal Septum

A deviated septum is an acceptable anatomical anomaly. The vast majority of people do not have symmetrical nasal septi but many ear, nose and throat specialists seize on this asymmetry as a reason to surgically correct a benign situation.

Radiation Causes Cancer

Madam Curie, who helped develop radium for cancer treatment, died of leukemia. This shows that radiation is very dangerous and should be used cautiously.

Unnecessary X-Rays

It has been estimated that up to one-third of all diagnostic X-rays are unnecessary.

Half-Life

The average individual is unaware of what the term half-life means when it is applied to synthetic chemical material introduced into the body. For example, when radioactive nuclear material, such as isotopes, are used for diagnostic purposes, half-life means the amount of time it takes for these isotopes to be reduced by one-half. If a substance has a half-life of 12 hours, every 12 hours its activity is reduced by one-half. Mathematically, that means there is always a residual amount of the substance remaining in the body.

Self-Fulfilling Prophesy

If a doctor says a patient has six months to live, that patient's participation in the treatment is decreased by his or her belief. In contrast to this, holistic physicians treat as if the patient will never die. Telling patients they have a limited time to live often becomes a self-fulfilling prophesy.

Photosensitivity

Some medications cause photosensitivity, and sunburn can occur even while using a sunscreen. The following may cause this:

- Certain heart medications
- Retin A
- Certain antibiotics, especially tetracyclines
- Birth control pills.

Medications Impair Driving Skills

People who are on certain medications are as much a menace on the highway as recreational drug addicts and alcoholics. The *Townsend Letter for Doctors,* June 1994, lists 225 prescription drugs that carry the warning, "Patients should be cautious not to operate dangerous machinery or a motor vehicle while taking this medicine."

Some of the more common medications in this category are:

- Actifed—for coughs
- Anaprox—non steroid anti-inflammatory
- Fiorinal with codeine—for migraine headaches

- Lasix—a diuretic
- Hycodan—cough remedy
- Hydrochlorothiazide—blood pressure medication
- Minocin—antibiotic
- Pamelor—antidepressant
- Tussi organidin—cough remedy
- Xanax—to treat anxiety attacks

Fluorine = Poison

Children living in areas where water is fluoridated, compared to those living in areas where water is not fluoridated, show no difference in the amount of dental cavities. In order for fluorine to be effective against tooth decay, it has to be applied directly to the teeth. Supplements of this material are ineffective and dangerous and can cause bladder cancer.

The need for fluorine in the body has never been demonstrated. In fact, fluorine binds up calcium and other essential minerals. Calcium is beneficial as an antidote for overdoses of fluorine. Latest studies show rats on fluorine had a much higher incidence of osteocarcinoma (bone cancer) than a control group. The rate of osteocarcinoma in humans was six to eight times higher in fluoridated areas and fluoridation has been abandoned throughout Europe.

The manufacture of aluminum or fertilizer and any coal-burning industry produces tons of fluorine as a waste product. Since it is difficult to dispose of, the industries found a viable market to rid themselves of a dangerous byproduct and add to their profit without regard to the cost of human suffering. Fluorine is much more toxic than lead and the one part per million in our drinking water leaches lead out of the pipes in the home, adding to the rise in lead levels in the body.

The Doctor Is Not Always Right

Most people have blind faith in the medical profession and believe the doctor is always right. However, this is not necessarily so. In fact, certain medications should never have been prescribed and certain procedures should never have been performed. For example:

- **DES**, prescribed to prevent miscarriages, caused cervical, vaginal and testicular cancer in the offspring of the women who took the drug.

- **Thalidamide**, used to alleviate nausea in pregnancy, resulted in birth deformities.
- **Tonsillectomies** weaken the immune system and leave scar tissue which harbors bacteria.
- **Halcion**, a sedative, causes amnesia and personality changes.
- **Swine flu vaccine**, given to elderly persons to protect them, in some cases actually caused the disease.
- **Milk used to treat stomach ulcers** has now been found as a possible cause of them.
- **IUD's** act as a wick to allow bacteria to enter the uterus.
- **Birth control pills**, as originally formulated, were found to contain too much estrogen and may have caused countless cases of uterine cancer.
- **Margarine**, touted for years as better than butter and lower in fat, has been scientifically proven to have caused heart attacks due to its transfatty acid composition.

3 Orthodox Propaganda

You Don't Have To Live With It!

The statement by orthodox physicians that patients must live with their disease for the rest of their lives is totally untrue. In fact, not explaining to the patient that there are other therapeutic methods for the improvement of their condition is a form of malpractice. No one should be expected to have to live with pain just because the medical establishment does not believe in other systems. Alternative methods used successfully in Europe have been kept out of the United States because the pharmaceutical companies fear competition.

The Enigma Of Hypoglycemia

Hypoglycemia is not a disease that needs medication. Since the pharmaceutical companies do not benefit from it, the medical establishment states that it is non-existent. Hypoglycemia causes blood sugar to drop drastically. This phenomenon, called low blood sugar, causes panic attacks and fatigue. In extreme cases, coma can occur. Complementary physicians believe hypoglycemia is a diet-related disease and can be eliminated by merely changing one's eating habits.

Government Misleads Public

Don't believe everything the government tells you. Interpretations of studies released to the public can be misleading. Case in point —The Tuskeegee Experiment in Alabama in the 30's. African-American men who had contracted syphilis were told they would be treated with certain medications that would cure their disease. In reality they were not given medication and studies were performed to see what would happen to patients not receiving treatment. This is immoral and demonstrates that some government agencies do not care if the patients live or die, but are only interested in furthering their knowledge of a disease, regardless of the consequence to the patient.

Freedom Of Choice

When a cancer patient seeks a second opinion from another doctor, chances are it will be the same as the first opinion since the orthodoxy has only three methods of treating the disease—surgery, chemotherapy or radiation. They do not recognize alternative therapy and are therefore doing the patient an injustice by not offering a true second opinion. Patients should have freedom to choose other treatments outside the realm of the orthodoxy.

Media Misleads Public

Informational programs about cancer on radio or television promote only orthodox treatment, with almost total disregard for prevention. This is another example of ignoring patients' well-being.

Doctors's Blunders—A Top Ten (Plus) Of Diagnosis Errors

- All high blood pressure requires medication.
- AIDS is a death sentence, in every case.
- Heart disease is irreversible.
- A low fat diet lowers cholesterol.
- Chronic fatigue syndrome is not real.
- Vaccinations are necessary for all children.
- There is no value in taking Vitamin C for the common cold.
- Diet has no effect on acne.
- Diet has no effect on colitis.
- All overweight people should be on a low fat diet.
- Sugar is not bad for hyperactive children with Attention Deficit Disorder. (ADD).
- Any sentence beginning with, "There is no proof."
- Low blood sugar is rare.

- There is no Candida syndrome.
- Food allergy is rare.
- Diabetics should be on a low fat, high carbohydrate diet.
- The only treatment for occluded coronary arteries is an angioplasty or bypass surgery.
- Ozone therapy has no clinical value.
- Chelation therapy has no clinical value.
- Diet has no effect on Crohn's Disease.

ALL WRONG!

Public Well-Being Ignored

Palm oil and coconut oil, beneficial oils, were driven off the market by the soybean oil conglomerate. The food industry has set nutrition policy in this country, disregarding the health hazards it imposes on the public.

Part II

Information on Conditions and Ailments

4 AIDS

HIV Positive Is Not Necessarily A Death Sentence

Only three percent of the population diagnosed HIV positive show signs of any symptoms.

Condoms

Despite what authorities tell our children, condoms are only 69 percent effective for the prevention of AIDS. The only way to protect yourself 100 percent from AIDS is not to have sex. However, those individuals with highly effective immune systems are protected from the ravages of viruses and bacteria from their sexual partners.

Vaccine

Hepatitis B vaccine is genetically engineered (produced from chemicals in a laboratory) rather than made from dead viruses. This makes it less likely to cause an allergic reaction. Individuals who are sexually active with multiple partners should be immunized against Hepatitis B which is a precursor to AIDS.

Dangers Of Orthodox Treatment

AZT is a chemotherapy agent that was used without success 20 years ago for cancer treatment. AZT destroys the immune system. Toxicology data clearly show the stem cells in the bone marrow are permanently damaged through the use of AZT.

DDI destroys the central nervous system. Side effects of DDI can cause pancreatitis, neurological disorders and liver damage.

Alpha-interferon used in the treatment of terminal diseases

such as AIDS is only 40 percent effective and causes disabling flu-like side effects.

AZT and DDI are used too early and in too high a dosage. Combining these with natural therapies enhances their effectiveness.

So-called HIV Positive individuals who felt well and were convinced to take AZT to kill the virus, eventually died from the medicine, not AIDS. Prior to taking AZT, these patients had no biochemical activity such as fever, high sedimentation rate, high white cell count, low red blood count, low platelet count or abnormal liver function tests, indicating that they did not, in effect, have AIDS. AZT is the most toxic drug ever devised by man. It is one of the worst forms of chemotherapy. It terminates DNA synthesis (destroys the function of the cell). AZT studies, known to be falsified, had been accepted by two government agencies who took them at their face value without investigation. Note—all patients on AZT eventually die.

National magazines with articles about AZT include *Science* April 9, 1993, *Time* April 12, 1993, *National Review* May 10, 1993 and *Business Week* July 26, 1993.

Magic Mushrooms

Three types of mushrooms are effective for the treatment of AIDS. Shiitake, Maitake and Reishi mushrooms stimulate the immune system. They can be consumed as food or are available in capsule form.

Ozone Therapy

Ozone sterilizes and purifies the blood. Ozone therapy can successfully treat AIDS, but the United States government suppresses its use. This treatment has had tremendous success rates in Europe, yet American physicians who utilize this therapy are subject to loss of license and jail sentences. As a case in point, Dr. James Boyce in Mississippi treated 113 AIDS patients and converted their blood from sera positive for AIDS to sera negative. No orthodox doctor has ever converted blood from sera positive to sera negative in an AIDS patient. Dr. Boyce was sentenced to jail.

Suppression Of Non-Toxic Treatment

The reasons ozone therapy is not widely offered are:

1. Large institutions which rely on sustaining grants for the scientific study of AIDS would lose their funding.

2. Pharmaceutical companies cannot patent ozone since it is a natural substance and is in the public domain. This is similar to the comment of a noted consumer advocate who said that solar energy would not be widely available until the utility companies could figure out a way to put a meter on the sun.

Patient's Right To Freedom Of Choice

AIDS patients, like cancer patients, do not have freedom of choice in selecting a non-toxic therapy that has been proven successful. Instead, they are given medications which actually exacerbate the problem by further depleting the immune system. AIDS patients seeking ozone therapy can obtain it in Europe or Mexico if they can't locate a local practitioner who has not been prosecuted.

Deadly Vaccine

AIDS could have been caused by a batch of contaminated vaccine (either polio or hepatitis vaccine).

Antibodies And AIDS

Diseases, with the exception of syphilis, Lyme disease and AIDS, are destroyed by the immune system's natural ability to produce antibodies. The first time a specific virus or bacteria enters the body, it is attacked by the body's immune system. In most cases the invader is destroyed and coded so the body will recognize it, if it attacks again, and overpower it with the previously-produced antibodies.

Since the immune system does not produce antibodies in cases of syphilis, Lyme disease and AIDS, there is no way for the body to defend itself. Therefore, antibiotics for syphilis and anti-viral medications for AIDS must be administered.

Note: AIDS is one of the few diseases where the virus attacks the immune system leaving no chance for it to defend itself.

False Positive HIV

Flu vaccine can cause a false positive HIV reading.

5 Alcoholism

Not Entirely A Psychological Problem

Alcoholism rehabilitation centers that do not use biological/ nutritional programs and rely solely on psychotherapy and medication, have a failure rate of almost 90 percent. Alcoholism is not entirely a psychological problem, but is often a biological one due to low insulin production which causes low blood sugar. The craving for alcohol replaces the need for sugar.

Allergic Reaction To Alcohol

Alcoholics are allergic to alcohol just as a person could be allergic to strawberries. The allergic reaction in alcoholics is the stimulus for them to drink alcohol. This fact is never addressed in the majority of alcohol rehabilitation centers which are more concerned with psychological therapy than with addressing this one biological cause of the disease.

Alcoholics have allergic reactions to wheat. Most alcoholic drinks are derived from grain. Rye whiskey is from wheat. Beer is from barley malt. Gin is from juniper berries. Vodka is from wheat or potatoes.

Sugar Craving

Although alcoholics may have stopped drinking, they are not well because they still crave large amounts of sugar. This craving for sugary foods replaces the craving for the sugar derived from alcohol, which is the initial problem.

Liver Dysfunction

Due to a deficiency of certain enzymes, alcoholics metabolize alcohol in their livers differently than other healthy people. The liver can be strengthened by the use of milk thistle (silymarin), dandelion root, and lipotropic factors (choline, inositol and methionine).

Hangovers

Conjuners are the hangover-causing substances in alcoholic drinks. Some beverages contain more than others. The highest concentrations are found in bourbon, brandy, red wine, rum and whiskey. Lower amounts are present in white wine and gin, and are virtually nonexistent in highly distilled vodka, which may be the drink of choice for those sensitive to conjuners.

Dehydration

Alcohol is a diuretic. It squeezes water out of the cells.

Herbal Remedy

Kudzu (an herb) alleviates the craving for alcohol.

Alcoholism On Campus

Forty percent of college students are considered binge drinkers.

Alcohol In Herbal Extracts

Anyone concerned about the alcohol in herbal extracts can remove the alcohol by adding the extract to a cup of boiling hot water or tea. Let the water cool before drinking it. Alcohol evaporates at a temperature of 170 degrees.

One Drink A Day

Alcohol in low doses (one drink a day) acts as a blood thinner.

6 Allergies

Grass Allergy

Sugar cane is a form of grass. If you have a grass allergy, you may also be allergic to sugar cane. In its place, use sugar made from beets or fruits.

Self-Testing

A simple test to determine environmental or food allergies is to take your pulse before eating a particular food or entering a specific area. Take it again 20 minutes later and, if it increases by 10 or more points, an allergy may be present.

Ragweed's Cousin

The protein in ragweed responsible for allergies is also present in melons and could cause an allergic reaction in susceptible individuals.

Food Allergy Self-Testing

When performing natural testing for food allergies, eat only brown rice and clarified butter for three days. This clears the body of all undigested food. Then add one food at a time and see if an allergic reaction occurs. Wait at least three hours between new food additions.

Allergic Reactive Foods

People who get a lot of allergic reactions to food should limit their diet to the following: lamb, chicken, potatoes, rice, bananas, pears, cucumbers, cabbage, celery, carrots, cauliflower, Brussels sprouts and broccoli.

Repetitive Dining

Most older people have food allergies because they frequently eat the same foods day after day. It is important to vary the diet.

Try Something New

People who are highly allergic to most foods often find they have no allergic reaction when changing to foods they have never eaten. The chance of an allergic reaction to the new food is minimal.

Self-Desensitization

Autogenis (a serum made from your own blood to desensitize you against allergic reactions) is not performed in the United States because of FDA regulations. In Europe it has been proven very successful.

Avoiding Pollen

The atmosphere is most heavily saturated with pollen and allergic materials between 5 and 10 am. Allergic people should avoid drying clothing outside as pollen clings to towels and sheets. Even though it is not the best thing for the atmosphere, drying clothing in an electric dryer is actually healthier for these people.

Histamine Blockers

Quercetin, a bioflavanoid, Vitamin C, and nettles block the release of histamine from the mast cells.

Oxygen Enhancement

Allergic reactions to food or airborne pollutants and pollens cause an acid condition in the body which can be alleviated by taking sodium bicarbonate to alkalinize the body. This process produces more oxygen which is needed to keep the blood vessels dilated, allowing more blood to flow to the reactive cells and decrease the histamine effect. Use one teaspoon of sodium bicarbonate to eight ounces of water twice daily or take Alka Seltzer Gold.

Symptoms In Children

Signs of allergies in children are red ear lobes, bright red cheeks, wiggly legs, rubbing the nose and making clicking throat sounds. They could be allergic to food or such environmental factors as molds, dust, synthetic carpet, deodorizers, disinfectants and aerosol sprays.

Yeast As A Cause Of Hives

A yeast problem can cause hives. If allergy tests are negative and the patient still has hives, he or she should be investigated for an overproliferation of yeast, which may be causing the allergy.

Decongestant Nasal Sprays

Do not use decongestant nasal sprays. They work temporarily and then cause a rebound effect which makes the allergy even worse.

Cats

If you are allergic to cats, you do not have to get rid of your pet. Just bathe the cat weekly to get rid of dander, which is usually the cause of the allergy.

Filters

The best filter to remove allergic debris in the house is an electrostatic filter.

Gas Stove

Asthma can be triggered by the fumes from a gas stove.

Niacin

People who are allergic should not use niacin (B^3) since it causes an increase in the amount of histamine released from the mast cells. Histamine is the byproduct of the allergic reaction and also has damaging effects on the liver.

7 Arthritis

Preserving The Cartilage

Osteoarthritis in the joints is caused by the drying up of the synovial fluid there. The cartilage wears out from this lack of lubrication and this causes the ends of the bones to rub together, which leads to severe pain and inflammation. This process can be slowed down by adding essential fatty acids to the diet. These fatty acids are found in animal food or supplements such as fish oil, cod liver oil, evening primrose oil or borage oil. Glucosamine sulfate, found in health food stores, is a precursor to cartilage.

Shark Cartilage

The latest testing shows that collagen from the breast bone of chickens is effective in treating rheumatoid arthritis. Yet, shark cartilage has been shown through many scientific studies to do the same thing at much lower cost, but it is not prescribed by medical doctors.

Therapeutic Mushrooms

Reishi mushrooms are effective as an anti-inflammatory for arthritis. In fact, they have a more powerful effect than prednisone without the harmful side effects.

Bee Venom Injections

Bee venom injections can reduce the inflammation of arthritis. Bee keepers do not contract arthritis since they are stung over a period of years and build up an immunity to most inflammatory joint problems. Caution—this therapy should not be used for people allergic to bee stings. Contact a practitioner in your area who has had experience with bee sting therapy.

Vegetarian Diet

An uncooked vegetarian diet helps rheumatoid arthritis sufferers.

Nightshades

Solanine, a chemical produced from plants in the nightshade family, including tomatoes, potatoes, bell peppers, eggplant and tobacco, is partly responsible for calcium being taken out of the bones and deposited in the joints where it causes inflammation and arthritic conditions. This is why arthritis sufferers are advised to avoid the nightshades.

Medication Is Merely Symptomatic Treatment

Medication for rheumatoid arthritis merely alleviates pain. As the disease continues, even more is prescribed, and eventually joint replacement is recommended. Cayenne red pepper salve, an over-the-counter item, can be applied topically to inflamed arthritic joints with highly positive results.

Bugs In Your Joints

Latest studies show that many people who have rheumatoid arthritis also have a systemic parasitic infection. This can be alleviated by a course of antibiotic therapy.

Buffering Zone

Too much protein in the diet leads to an acidic condition of the body so the body tries to buffer this condition by drawing calcium from the blood and transporting it to inflamed acidic sites, usually the joints. During this process, some of the calcium stays in the joint as calcium deposits and these eventually lead to immobility and the wearing down of the cartilage which causes pain and further inflammation. This process can be stopped by taking potassium bicarbonate or Alka Seltzer Gold to alkalinize the system.

Arthritis-Digestion Connection

Bacteria in your digestive tract can cause arthritis. Colon cleansing or intestinal balancing with acidophilus can help. Your diet should be wheat-free and gluten products should be eliminated. Meat contains arachidonic acid which causes inflammation and should also be avoided.

Don't Drink The Water

Fluorine, which has been added to most municipal water supplies to strengthen teeth and bones, causes bone growth in arthritic joints. Drink steam-distilled water only.

An Omelet For Arthritis

Foods with a high sulfur content help remove metallic deposits from the system. Eggs, asparagus, garlic and onions are high in sulfur.

Check Your Multi-Vitamin

If you are taking a multi-vitamin, be sure it does not contain iron, which can cause pain, swelling, production of free radicals and destruction of your joints.

8 Asthma

Blow Up A Balloon

If you have a respiratory condition, such as asthma, emphysema and bronchitis, you can strengthen your lungs by blowing up a balloon 40 times through the course of a day.

Swimming

Swimming is a good exercise for asthmatics because the air is moist and because they have to practice breath control. It is one of the very few exercises that actually *increases* lung volume.

Diaphragmatic Breathing Exercise

This exercise strengthens the muscles around your lung.

In a sitting position, place hands on lower abdomen. Exhale completely through mouth while pushing on your abdomen, at the same time contracting the abdominal muscles.

Breathe in through nose until your hands on your abdomen separate. Hold breath to a count of 10. Repeat 10 times.

Expectorant

A few drops of potassium iodide in water is an effective expectorant that helps to clear mucous from the lungs.

Hot Pepper

Hot pepper (cayenne) loosens mucous in asthmatics and helps to open up the blood vessels and allow more oxygen to enter the lungs.

Beware Of Cold Air

Asthmatics who exercise outdoors in cold weather should use a mask over their noses and mouths to keep inhaled air warm.

Cold Shower

Take a cold shower to relieve an asthma attack.

Water Cure

Drinking three quarts of water daily will relieve asthma because water in large amounts interrupts histamine production.

Test For Lung Problems

To test for lung problems, such as asthma, bronchitis and emphysema, hold a lighted match at arm's length and try to blow it out. If you have to bring it within six inches of your face to blow it out, you have a lung problem.

Latex Sensitivity

People with asthma are often allergic to latex products which could precipitate an asthmatic attack. They should be wary of coming into contact with latex materials such as condoms, gloves and diaphragms.

Up In Smoke

Of the nearly one million new smokers last year, most were children. This early consumption of tobacco is the main reason why more children are contracting asthma.

N.A.C. Expectorant

N.A.C. (N. Acetyl Cysteine, an amino acid), 600 mg four times daily is a useful expectorant for asthma patients.

Magnesium Deficiency

Latest studies show asthmatic patients may have a magnesium deficiency. Supplementing with 500 mg of magnesium citrate or magnesium aspartate three times daily will help relax muscle spasms. If diarrhea occurs, cut back the dosage.

9 Bowels

Parasites

Patients with Chron's disease, colitis or irritable bowel syndrome should be checked for parasites. They may be the culprits.

Parasite Remedy

To treat parasites, use artemesia, grapefruit seed extract, black walnut hulls, goldenseal and Paramicrociden.

Too Many Tests

People with irritable bowel syndrome, colitis and Chron's Disease receive too many tests from medical doctors which do not usually show a cause for the disease. The doctors, in their befuddlement, continue to put the patients through even more uncomfortable invasive testing when the real cause for these conditions is often merely an intestinal reaction to certain foods. Yet, patients are hardly ever asked about their diets and are usually told to eat whatever they like, and so the condition gets worse. These people should be investigated for food allergy. If this is done first, it would be more cost-effective and the patient could be spared a lot of discomfort.

Bowel Balance

Bran and whole wheat products are detrimental to patients with irritable bowel syndrome. Soluble soft fiber should be used instead. Good sources of soluble fiber are apple pectin, lignan and guar gum products.

Traveler's Aid

If you are traveling in third world countries, take two Pepto-Bismol tablets four times daily. This will protect you from diarrhea and unfamiliar disease-causing organisms. Note: A temporary darkening of the stool may occur but this is no cause for alarm.

Flaxseed

The best remedy for constipation is flaxseed (the seeds, not the oil or capsules). Flaxseed can be added to cereals and breads or sprinkled on salads.

The Bowel/Sinus Connection

Too much mucous in the bowel can cause sinus inflammation. Cleansing the bowels often relieves congestion in other parts of the body.

Honey For Diarrhea

Due to its low water content and its ability to absorb water from the colon, raw honey is useful in controlling diarrhea. An excess of water in the colon activates the urge to have a bowel movement.

Diet For Diarrhea

To stop diarrhea, eat a high protein, low carbohydrate diet.

Diarrhea Remedy

Calcium lactate pills can control diarrhea. It is also helpful to convert the body's pH from acid to alkaline by taking bicarbonate of soda or Alka Seltzer Gold.

Constipation Remedy

Aloe vera capsules are an effective remedy for constipation.

Puréed Food

Individuals with inflammatory bowel disease should limit their diet to puréed food when the condition is active. Put all food into a blender or a food processor.

Nicotine Patch For Ulcerative Colitis

Transdermal nicotine patches were shown to improve ulcerative colitis by 25 percent compared with a placebo group. This does not mean patients who suffer from this should take up smoking since cigarettes contain many harmful chemicals. Used this way (via patches), nicotine has positive pharmaceutical effects and avoids the damaging side effects of carbon dioxide, formaldehyde, tar and nitrosamines that are associated with smoking it. The patches are pure nicotine.

Detoxifiers

Apple pectin, guar gum and alginate, available in health food stores, act as detoxifiers because they absorb toxins and heavy metals in the colon.

After The Cleaning

Colon cleansing is sometimes necessary to get rid of debris that has clung to the sides of the colon and is causing inflammation and blocking the absorption of specific nutrients. After colon cleansing (a high colonic), you must replace the friendly bacterial cultures (acidophilus) that were also flushed out. These cultures provide hydrogen peroxide which acts as the body's natural free radical scavenger.

10 Cancer

Losing The War

The war on cancer is somewhere between a disappointment and an outright failure. In 1900, the death rate from cancer was three percent. It is now 22 percent. Statistics from the National Cancer Institute show, after 23 years and $35 billion in research, that no appreciable decrease in the age-adjusted incidence of cancer has been demonstrated. The death rate is up seven percent and the five-year survival rate is virtually unchanged.

Cancer Is On The Rise

JAMA (*Journal of the American Medical Association*) February 9, 1994 states: The bad news is that the incidence of cancer is increasing in all age groups in the United States, and that few new effective treatments have been found for the most common cancers.

Current Technology Inadequate

After years of observing patients, I have come to the conclusion that people diagnosed with cancer do not actually have true cancer. They may, indeed, have tumors, but a large percent of them are benign, not malignant.

I am not stating that the doctors are lying to the public maliciously, but current scientific technology does not allow us to see the portion of the cell which determines whether the patient will survive and return to normal health.

How Cancer Starts

Ask any orthodox doctor how a cancer got started and the answer is, "We don't know." In actuality, the flood of chemicals in our food, air and water causes changes to the DNA in the body's cells leading to the abnormal growth of tissues which can become cancerous. For example, when a factory discharges its liquid wastes into a river, the fish eventually develop cancerous livers and die. Next the foliage surrounding the river dies and eventually the people living near the river contract cancer.

Cancer And EMF

A Swedish study showed a rise in childhood leukemia in children living in homes close to transformers and high tension wires that emit electromagnetic fields.

EMF's Kill

Males exposed to electromagnetic fields are contracting breast cancer up to six times the expected rate. Women exposed to electromagnetic fields are dying from all cancers 40 percent more than those not exposed. Leukemia is also higher in children exposed to these EMF's. Magnetic fields suppress melatonin production, and melatonin protects against breast cancer.

Chlorinated Chemicals Poison Females

Estrogenic factors (xeno estrogens) are derived from chlorinated chemicals such as DDT, PCB and other pesticides, and exacerbate cancer in female organs by stimulating the estrogens in the ovaries.

Driving Can Be Dangerous To Your Health

Catalytic converters required in automobiles are made from platinum which permeates the driver's area and can cause adenocarcinoma of the lungs. Be sure the car is well ventilated and drive with windows slightly open at all times.

Danger From Your Faucet

Studies have shown that men who drink tap water contract more bladder cancer than men who drink bottled water.

Beware Of Ultrasound

Ultrasound can intensify the growth of cancer cells.

Radiology, A Dangerous Profession

Leukemia is 1000 times more common for radiologists than for all other physicians combined.

Lack Of Oxygen Sabotages Cells

Any organ depleted of enough oxygen will reverse its biological system to a plant-like biology which thrives off fermentation in order to obtain oxygen from other substances. This process causes the cell to convert from a biological human cell to a plant-type cell which can eventually become carcinogenic.

Sweet Death

Intravenous glucose administered to cancer patients hastens the disease because cancer is an anaerobic disease which thrives on sugar and lives without oxygen. Too much sugar in the blood reduces the amount of oxygen available to the cells, causing them to deteriorate further.

Low Potassium Levels Invite Cancer

A cell containing a normal amount of potassium will not overgrow and eventually become a tumor because potassium activates enzymes which protect the cell. If the cell is too low in sodium, it will also be too low in potassium, so salt-free diets are not necessarily the best ones for you.

Stay Away From Iron

Latest studies show that the more iron there is in the blood, the greater the risk of esophageal and bladder cancer.

Stress Feeds Cancer

Stress causes the endocrine gland system to release cortisol and prolactin, two substances which stimulate the growth of cancer cells.

The Pill May Be Dangerous To Your Health

Oral contraceptives may cause cervical cancer if they are used for several years.

Inconsiderate Doctors

Stress caused by an extended wait for mammogram results could lower the immune system enough to allow the formation of cancer cells. It seems to me that doctors who make patients wait so long for test results are not taking the patients' peace of mind into consideration.

Green Tea And Mushrooms

Green tea and maitake mushrooms are immune system enhancers and are particularly effective in warding off cancer.

Tuna Is A Girl's Best Friend

Tuna fish is high in selenium, a nutrient that is important in protecting women from breast cancer.

A Bean A Day Keeps Breast Cancer Away

Soy products contain phytoestrogens which can protect against breast cancer. Beans also contain high amounts of this substance. Fish oil contains prostaglandins, which are precursors to anti-inflammatory hormones and also protect against breast cancer and other inflammatory diseases.

Exercise And Cancer

Moderate exercise increases the number of beneficial killer cells. Excessive exercise, however, can be counterproductive because it produces free radicals which have a harmful effect on the immune system.

Exercise Stymies Cancer

Women who exercise have one-sixteenth the cancer risk of sedentary women. Men who exercise have one-quarter the cancer risk of sedentary men.

Beware Of The B Vitamins

B vitamins are growth promoters. Therefore it's not a good idea for cancer patients to overdo on high amounts of the B's.

Thwart X-Ray Effects

X-rays have an ionizing effect that is dangerous. They cause cells to mutate, a precursor to cancer. If X-rays are unavoidable, take high amounts of Vitamin C, glutathione, and N.A. cysteine for one week and drink large amounts of distilled water.

Moving To America Can Be Bad For Your Health

If nutritional factors are not important, why do so many Japanese contract cancer when they change their diets after moving to the United States mainland?

Japanese Diet Wins War

Phytoestrogens (natural plant estrogens from soy, tofu, alfalfa and pomegranates) block the overproduction of an overactive type of male and female hormones. This may be a reason for the low incidence of uterine, ovarian, breast and prostate cancer in Japan.

Veggies That Zap Female Cancers

Soy products, beans, and vegetables in the cabbage family contain chemicals (indoles) that naturally block the type of estrogen that can cause cancer in females.

Healthy Beverages

Polyphenols, plant extracts found in red wine and green tea, protect the body from free radicals and cancer.

Unhealthy Beverages

According to the latest studies, chemicals in tap water may cause bladder cancer. Drink distilled water or use a quality filter.

Starve The Tumor

Cancer patients should eliminate animal protein in order to starve the cancerous tumors which depend on protein. In this case, a vegetarian diet is appropriate.

Friendly Fats

All fats are not equal. Fats from meats, poultry and dairy products may cause cancer, while fats from fish reduce the likelihood of contracting cancer.

Butter Your Bread

Butyric acid (butyrate), found in butter, is very effective in treating leukemia.

Veggies Stymie Cancer

The same biological chemicals in certain plants that protect them against fungi and insects also protect human beings against cancer. These plants, in the cruciferous and carotenoid families, are broccoli, Brussels sprouts, cabbage, carrots and most other yellow and orange vegetables.

Cabbage For Your Health

Indoles in cabbage will help bond estrogens in the body, keeping them from going to possible cancerous sites that are estrogen dependent.

Go Macrobiotic

A macrobiotic diet is very effective in the treatment of prostate or uterine cancer.

The Best Cancer

Thyroid cancer is the least malignant and has the lowest chance of spreading.

Eighty-Seven Percent Death Rate

Lung cancer has only a 13 percent cure rate.

Conventional Treatment For Pancreatic Cancer Fails

Ninety-five percent of pancreatic cancer patients treated by conventional methods are dead within a year. Patients with pancreatic cancer could consult Dr. Robert Atkins, who is having excellent results, and Dr. Nicholas Gonzales of Manhattan has had an 85 percent remission rate if his treatment is strictly followed.

Understand The Diagnosis

Undifferentiated carcinoma means that the boundaries of the cancer have extended and the primary cancer site is unknown.

Mole Identification

The ABCD's used to identify a mole as cancerous are:

A — Asymmetry
B — Border is irregular
C — Change of color
D — Diameter is larger than 6 mm.

It is important to seek medical attention if any or all of these markers are evident.

Breast Cancer On The Rise

In 1950, one of every 20 women contracted breast cancer. In 1990 one of every eight women contracted breast cancer.

Deceptive Statistics

The statement that one of every eight women will contract breast cancer is deceptive. One in eight is a lifetime incidence of breast cancer. At age 40, the probability is one in 217; at age 50, one in 50. After age 50, the probability escalates rapidly, but breast cancer does not grow as fast or spread as rapidly in older women.

Family History

Most women who contract breast cancer do not have a family history of the disease.

Breast Cancer Factors

Women on estrogen replacement therapy for five years stand a 50 percent higher chance of contracting breast cancer. Women on oral contraceptives for five years have a 15 percent higher chance. Women over five feet, nine inches tall have an 80 percent higher chance of acquiring breast cancer.

Keep Progesterone Levels Up

Women with low progesterone levels are 10 times more likely to contract cancer.

Another Breast Cancer Risk

Women who have had an abortion stand a greater chance of developing breast cancer.

Testosterone Levels

Breast cancer in older women may be caused by low testosterone levels, not high estrogen.

Breast-Feeding Benefits Mothers Too

Mothers who breast-feed their infants reduce their chance of contracting breast cancer by 20 percent before menopause. This is because ovulation is interrupted.

Mammograms Not 100 Percent Reliable

Ten to 15 percent of all breast cancers will not be detected on a mammogram. A cancerous breast lump feels like a pebble or a stone.

Mammograms

Mammograms do not prevent cancer. They diagnose it if it is already present, and it is often too late.

Mammograms Unreliable For Young Women

Mammography is not an effective diagnostic tool for premenopausal women as their breast tissue is quite dense, which makes it difficult to differentiate between diseased and normal tissue.

Mammograms Miss

Fifteen percent of breast cancers do not show on a mammogram.

Estrogen/Breast Cancer Connection

There is a higher incidence of breast cancer in places where high rates of estrogen are prescribed.

Timing Crucial For Breast Cancer Surgery

Breast cancer surgery should not be performed during a woman's ovulatory phase because, if the cancer is estrogen receptive, the outcome would be more successful when less estrogen is being produced.

Tamoxifen

Tamoxifen, used in the treatment of breast cancer following surgery, has been shown to cause endometrial dysplasia, a precancerous condition of the lining of the uterus.

Most Radiation Unnecessary Following Lumpectomy

Radiation after lumpectomy for post-menopausal women with negative, cancer-free lymph nodes is usually not necessary, but is often administered.

Radiation Fails To Zap Metastasis

Radiation for breast cancer has never been proven to prevent the spread of the cancer, but only shown to be partially effective against recurrences of cancer in the breasts themselves.

Radiation Damages Heart

Radiation to the chest area for breast cancer or lung cancer causes scarring which can damage the heart.

Chemotherapy Damages Heart

Adramiacin, a chemotherapeutic drug used to treat breast cancer, damages the heart.

Aid Lymphatic Drainage

To help lymphatic fluid drain from the arm of breast cancer patients who have had the lymph nodes in the armpit area removed, there is a device which uses pressure to force the fluid from the swollen lymph system. Massages also work. If these methods are not effective, it might indicate that cancer is still present and the patient should be re-evaluated.

Lymphedema Pumps

Most pumps for the relief of lymphedema (swelling of the arm after removal of lymph nodes in the armpit) following breast surgery do not work. In fact they can be counterproductive, often causing an undesirable tourniquet effect. Dr. Jacobs of Cooper Hospital in Camden, New Jersey says lymph pumps have to work sequentially with intermittent compression, starting from the hand up.

Flesh Foods Feed Cancer

Anyone with a predisposition to colon cancer should abstain from eating animal food. Bile, which is required for the digestion of animal food, can cause inflammation to the sides of the colon which may lead to the beginning of cancer.

Fiber In — Cancer Out

Vitamin C, along with a high fiber diet, converts cholesterol in the body to bile salts which are excreted through the colon, thereby lessening the possibility of colon cancer.

Fish Oil Slows Polyps

Fish oil supplements slow the growth of precancerous cells in colon polyps.

Colon Cancer Insurance

For protection against colon cancer, use selenium, calcium, folic acid, vitamins D, E and C, and eat a high fiber diet.

Folic Acid Prevents Colon Cancer

Folic acid administered to people with colitis reduces, by 50 percent, the chance of abnormally growing tissue turning malignant.

Watchful Waiting Fails

The statement that every male who lives long enough will develop prostate cancer is erroneous and it plants a seed in the patient's psyche which inevitably becomes a self-fulfilling prophesy. Doctors treating prostate cancer use the term "watchful waiting" which means nothing is done therapeutically while the tumor enlarges. Patients, in their ignorance of any method to deter the growth of the tumor, continue to follow the same lifestyle and therefore nothing is done to improve the situation.

Watchful Waiting OK For Older Males

Males age 60 and older with early prostate cancer were studied for two years using 3 different treatment methods (radiation, surgery and watchful waiting). No significant differences in remission rates were found. In older males with early prostate cancer, the cancer is slow-growing and doesn't spread rapidly.

Note: A very effective treatment for prostate cancer is a macrobiotic diet consisting of vegetables, soy products and sea vegetables.

Everything You Should Know About The PSA

Prostate cancer is very slow-growing in men over age 65. Even if rectal examination results and the PSA (prostate specific antigen, a blood test for cancer of the prostate) are abnormal, the patient may not necessarily have cancer. The PSA test should be considered an early warning system. Normal PSA readings range from 0 to 4. Readings ranging from 4 to 10 can indicate the presence of a malignancy confined to the prostate. If the readings are over 10, the cancer may have metastasized and an ultrasound rectally-guided biopsy should be performed.

If the reading rises by more than .75 of one increment of the four within a year, then cancer should be suspected and further investigation is needed. For example, if the original reading is 3.0 and it raises to 3.8 in a year, that is more than a .75 rise.

Know Your PSA Numbers

PSA readings of 18 or higher indicate prostate cancer is outside the gland and may have metastasized. A reading of 40 or above means the cancer is in the bones.

Timing The PSA

The PSA should be performed prior to a digital rectal examination which can inflame the prostate, causing a false high reading.

Prostate Volume Significant

When diagnosing prostate cancer using the PSA test, the weight and size of the prostate gland must also be taken into consideration. If the gland is enlarged, a PSA reading in the cancer range may not necessarily indicate a malignancy.

Unnecessary Surgery

Men over 70, with a PSA reading of 11, do not necessarily require surgery. It is only necessary to monitor them for urinary blockage.

PSA Often Unreliable

Twenty to 30 percent of men with prostate cancer have normal PSA test readings and 20 to 25 percent of PSA readings are false positive.

Needle Biopsy Can Miss Malignancy

With a high PSA reading, a negative needle biopsy does not necessarily eliminate the possibility of prostate cancer. Unless the needle is accurately guided to the cancerous area by a sonogram, the malignancy could be missed.

Prostate Exam

Eighty percent of prostate cancer occurs on the posterior surface of the prostate gland (the side toward the rectum) allowing the physician to easily feel an abnormality.

Unnecessary Castration

If an orchidectomy (removal of testicles) is performed to stop testosterone production in prostate cancer, it is only 90 percent effective since 10 percent of testosterone is produced in the adrenals. Flutamide, an antihormonal substance, is used to stop adrenal production of testosterone.

Nothing Is Better Than Something

Studies have shown that men over 60 with prostate cancer do just as well or better without treatment as men treated with surgery, radiation and chemotherapy.

Men Should Self-Exam

Just as women are taught to examine their own breasts, men should also be taught how to examine their testicles for any abnormalities that could be symptoms of testicular cancer.

Nix Chemotherapy For Prostate Cancer

Chemotherapy is never effective for prostate cancer, and should never be used.

Prostate Radiation Unwise

Radiation to the prostate inflames the mucous membrane of the colon and the bladder.

Irreversible Effects Of Prostate Radiation

Radiation to the prostate can cause scar tissue to form in the area. If further treatment with chemotherapy is necessary, the scar tissue will prevent it from being effective due to the destruction of circulation in that area. Radiation also depletes the immune system.

Non-Toxic Prostate Treatment

To treat prostate cancer in patients with high PSA readings, use Lupron or Ulexon (antihormonal medication) and localized hyperthermia (heat treatment produced by microwave frequency, generally through a probe inserted into the penis) in conjunction with the supplements glycine, glutamic acid, alanine, zinc, magnesium and saw palmetto berries. This combination which has minimal, if any, side effects can reduce a PSA as high as 70, which denotes cancer, down to 0 to 4, which are normal readings.

Prostate Surgery Not Indicated

Surgery is not indicated for prostate cancer since antihormonal medication in combination with alternative therapy is so effective.

Side Effects Of Antihormonal Drugs

A side effect of antihormonal drugs used in prostate cancer can be enlargement and lumps in men's breasts.

Go Macrobiotic

A macrobiotic diet for prostate cancer limits all animal food containing proteins that make the tumor grow. Prostate cancer is hormone-based and responds particularly well to diet.

Stay Clear Of Radiation

Radiation from the sun, computers, microwave ovens and other electromagnetic fields produces free radicals which change the DNA, setting the individual up for cancer. The treatment for many cancers is even more radiation in the form of X-ray therapy. The same radiation which causes the cancer is also used to treat the disease and can cause cancer in other parts of the body at a later date.

Radium Seeds

Radium seeds implanted directly at the cancerous site do less damage and are more effective than external radiation.

Cancer Reappears Following Radiation

Radiation can shrink tumors, but in many cases the tumor reappears in other areas of the body and is more virulent than the original one. This is called population genetics. The radiation destroys the least active cells and does not affect the most resistant mutated cells which then become more dangerous, causing cancer in another part of the body.

Radiation Hampers Future Treatment

Radiation destroys blood supply in body tissue. Therefore, chemotherapy or any other medication cannot be transported to the diseased area that was treated.

Hyperthermia And Radiation

Hyperthermia (raising body temperature) enhances the success rate of radiation therapy from 15 percent to 85 percent. Patients have fewer side effects and the amount of radiation can be reduced by one-half. Although this process is beneficial to cancer patients, the medical orthodoxy does not take advantage of it. Usually, the last 10 to 20 percent of radiation administered causes problems due to its cumulative effect.

Free Radical Cleanser

Cancer patients receiving radiation should take NAC (N. Acytl cysteine) to cleanse the body of free radicals formed from the radiation.

The Oncologist's Goal

Oncologists administering chemotherapy have only one goal, the destruction of the tumor. This goal is so paramount that the restoration of health is not even considered. Oncologists give a *response* rate, not a cure rate, which is confusing to the patient.

Response Rate

When an oncologist says chemotherapy or radiation is 15 to 20 percent effective, he or she is referring to the response rate, not the cure rate. Response rate applies to the shrinkage of a tumor for 28 days, without taking into consideration what happens after that period of time. This in no way equates with an increase in survival time. If the immune system is not continually stimulated by proper nutrition and supplementation, the cancer will eventually return.

Exercise In Futility

The three essential parameters to keep in mind when considering chemotherapy, radiation or surgery are:

1. Extension of life.
2. Quality of life
3. Shrinkage of the tumor.

Most orthodox practitioners stress tumor shrinkage rather than extension of, or quality of life. If all three cannot be guaranteed by the oncologist, undergoing this horrendous treatment is an exercise in futility.

Most Chemotherapy Unnecessary Following Lumpectomy

Studies show chemotherapy and/or radiation following lumpectomy does not extend life. This type of adjunctive therapy is effective in only 6 percent of patients, but is wrong 94 percent of the time. This grueling type of therapy causes hair loss, destruction of bone marrow, mouth ulcers, diarrhea, depression and unending fatigue. The $64,000 question is — Why isn't a determination made beforehand to give it only to the 6 percent who really need it? It is unfair to subject a human being to such torture for the financial rewards gleaned from the therapy that in most cases is not necessary.

Futility Of Chemotherapy

In certain cases, chemotherapy is warranted and may cause remission, but the side effects are horrendous and in later life cancers often form in other parts of the body due to depletion of the immune system.

While one of my patients was being treated with chemotherapy for a tumor in her descending colon, she developed an additional tumor in the ascending colon. This shows the futility of this type of therapy. With natural healing therapy, the disease went into remission, and she lived to a ripe old age with an excellent quality of life.

Chemotherapy Useless For Ovarian Cancer

The use of chemotherapy for ovarian cancer initiates a response rate, not a *cure* rate. The response rate is short-lived and the cancer recurs. The cure rate from chemotherapy for this type of cancer is zero, yet oncologists still prescribe this worthless pain-inflicting medication.

No Chemotherapy For Colon Cancer

Patients who receive chemotherapy following surgery for colon cancer fare only slightly better than those who do not. Yet, the doctors continue to use chemotherapy even though its side effects have disastrous effects on patients in such a weakened condition.

Chemotherapy Now — Cancer Later

Chemotherapy administered for one kind of cancer can lead to another type of cancer at a later date.

Unnecessary Chemotherapy

If lymph nodes near the primary site of a cancer are not positive, chemotherapy is not needed. Yet, it is usually recommended.

Antiquated Forms Of Chemotherapy

Chemotherapeutic cancer medications such as methotrexate, # 5 FU and cytoxin are outdated drugs which do not work well at all and cause many painful side effects.

Overused Chemotherapy

Chemotherapy is ineffective in colorectal cancer. Therefore it is not an appropriate treatment.

Ineffective Melanoma Treatment

Latest studies show chemotherapy is ineffective for treating melanoma.

Chemotherapy Shortens Lives

Latest studies show 30 percent of all patients taking chemotherapy had shortened lives and eventually died.

Chemotherapy Lowers Survival Rate

Each and every chemotherapy treatment drops the survival rate by four percent.

Chemotherapy's Side Effects Last

Side effects of chemotherapy continue long after treatment is over.

Bone Marrow Transplant

A bone marrow transplant is merely a way to rescue the body from the toxicity of the very high doses of chemotherapy given in cancer therapy.

Chemotherapy Antidote

Chemotherapy kills cancer cells. Then the dead cells produce poisons and the patient dies from the poisoning rather than from the original cancer. In order to avoid this, the dead cancer cells must be eliminated from the body by detoxification methods, such as coffee enemas and gallbladder flushes (olive oil therapy) and kidney flushes (drinking at least twelve eight ounce glasses of water daily, or until the urine is colorless).

Get Your Chemotherapy In Germany

Dr. Hans Neiper of Germany mixes chemotherapy with liposomes, a process which insures that the chemotherapy is delivered only to the cancerous tumor, thus sparing the normal cells.

Cancer Returns

Nodular lymphoma and most cancers usually recur in 2 years even when they are treated with chemotherapy and radiation.

Liver Therapy Ousts Lymphoma

Lymphoma recurs even though chemotherapy is used as a treatment. A more lasting, effective nutritional approach would be to strengthen the liver in order to allow it to cleanse the body of toxic materials, thereby lessening the load on the lymphatic system.

Keep Your Hair

To prevent hair loss during chemotherapy, use high doses of Vitamin E (2400 I.U.).

Squelch Chemotherapy's Side Effects

Since chemotherapy produces free radicals, it is essential to take antioxidants like Vitamins A, C, E, selenium and glutathione while undergoing this toxic treatment.

Marijuana — The Unused Pain Killer

One of the best ways to control nausea and pain due to chemotherapy is marijuana. Cancer patients are denied this while morphine is prescribed, eventually causing an addiction which can be worse than the original problem.

Antioxidants Save Cells

Cancer cells are more vulnerable to chemotherapy and radiation because they don't have antioxidant defenses. Normal cells have defenses against radiation, chemotherapy and the environment. Therefore the use of antioxidants like Vitamins A, C, E, selenium and glutathione while undergoing these procedures will help protect the normal cells.

Chemotherapy Is Bad For Your Health

Forty percent of cancer patients die from malnutrition, not the cancer. Chemotherapy leads to malnutrition by causing diarrhea, nausea, loss of appetite and poor circulation.

Nutrition For Chemotherapy Patients

Malnourishment, a side effect of chemotherapy, is due to the patient's inability to digest nutrients. Chemotherapy destroys all fast-growing cells, including those in the intestines where nutrients are absorbed. To receive proper nourishment, these patients should take pre-digested proteins, fats and carbohydrates such as Ensure. Vitamins should be used in the mycellized form. Mycellized vitamins are the fat soluble A, D and E vitamins which have their fat broken down to a smaller molecule for easier absorption by those who have difficulty digesting fats and oils.

Appetite Stimulator

Extremely debilitated cancer patients who have lost their appetite should be given hydrazine sulfate, an appetite enhancer. This is a prescription item.

High levels of progesterone do not cause cancer but can cause breakthrough bleeding in women. They can also increase the appetite. This side effect of increasing the appetite is useful in female terminal cancer patients who are debilitated from not eating.

Hi-Tech Overrated

Overall statistics show that the mortality and survival time for cancer patients has not changed in the past 20 years even though the National Institute of Health introduces new "so-called miraculous" cancer treatments on a yearly basis.

Public Lied To

When a major cancer hospital tested alternative and non-toxic treatments for cancer and found results were positive, the public affairs staff was instructed to report negative conclusions to the public. They made false statements, especially about Laetrile.

For more information, read *The Cancer Industry Or The Cancer Syndrome* by Ralph Moss. In cancer treatment, conventional methods are toxic while alternative treatments are non-toxic. The establishment refers to alternative treatments as quack treatments. Moss's book, *Cancer Therapy, The Independent Consumer's Guide To Non-toxic Treatment And Prevention* offers 100 treatments, whereas the orthodoxy offers only three: surgery, radiation and chemotherapy. Moss derived all his information from medical journals published since 1966. Ninety-six of these treatments are documented in peer review journals. More scientific justification exists for the use of non-toxic treatment in these journals than for the use of toxic treatment.

FDA Cancels Cancell

The FDA is more concerned with stopping alternative therapy than it is in patients' welfare. A case in point is the use of Cancell, an alternative treatment for cancer that was used successfully in treating 10,000 patients. The FDA stopped distribution of Cancell by citing interstate commerce regulations. These did not really apply since Cancell was being distributed at no charge. Since then, many people who were kept alive by Cancell have died unnecessarily. If the function of the FDA is to protect the public, why is it destroying so many people?

Establishment Ignores Effective Hormonal Treatment

DHEA is the precursor of male and female hormones. It is used by holistic physicians to treat cancer and stimulate the immune system. However, overdosing can cause the masculinizing of females who become aggressive, develop deeper voices and grow facial hair. DHEA should be administered only to the levels in the body at age 30. DHEA is in squalene (shark liver oil) and Mexican wild yams.

Shark Cartilage Saves Cubans

A Cuban study was performed using shark cartilage in the treatment of 29 terminal cancer patients with stage 4 cancer. These patients had undergone chemotherapy, radiation and surgery and were expected to die within six months. At the end of 25 months, 14 were completely well with no sign of cancer, six died of other ailments and nine died of the cancer.

Shark Cartilage Starves Most Cancers

Shark cartilage, while effective in treating many cancers, does not aid lymphoma or leukemia patients since these types do not have the same blood supply as a solid tumor, the type most cancers are. Shark cartilage works by cutting off the blood supply in the arteries that feed the tumor with blood and nutrients, especially sugars, which nourish tumors. It also has been shown to reverse metastasis to the bone.

Benefits Of Shark Cartilage

When taking shark cartilage, cancer patients often show:

- Enhanced quality of life in four to six weeks.
- Pain reduction in eight to ten weeks.
- Shrinkage of tumor in twelve weeks.

Cook Up Your Own Anti-Cancer Cocktail

ESSIAC, a formula developed by a Canadian nurse, Mrs. Caisse (Essiac spelled backwards), has been shown to be effective in cancer treatment. Studies on this formula performed by the Canadian government show a 95 percent remission rate in all types of cancer. The formula is as follows:

- 6 ½ cups burdock root
- 16 ounces sheep sorrel
- 1 ounce turkey rhubarb
- 4 ounces slippery elm bark

Mix all ingredients in a 5 gallon stainless steel container.
Fill container with hot water, and steep 5 minutes.
Drink 4 cups daily.

Cayce Cabbage Therapy

An Edgar Cayce remedy for breast cancer is to heat four to five cabbage leaves in a pan until the ends start to curl. Cool the leaves and wrap them around the breast for 24 hours. According to Cayce, this causes the cancer to be detoxified and then eliminated. The treatment can be repeated in another 24 hours.

Juice For Health

The Gerson Therapy is excellent for treating melanomas. It consists of juicing, one to five coffee enemas daily and specialized supplementation. This therapy works by balancing potassium within the cell with sodium outside of the cell. A transport system exists between the sodium and potassium, but if too much sodium infiltrates the cell, it will displace the potassium which is needed to protect the cell against viruses (cancer). For a more detailed explanation of how this works, read *Results of 50 Cases* by Max Gerson, M.D.

Immune System Stimulant

Cancer patients lose the ability to produce gamma inteferon (an immune system stimulant). Ginseng aids in the production of inteferon.

Awakening The Immune System

The Keef method used in Germany is a therapeutic procedure for the treatment of cancer. It uses the patient's own blood cells to seek out and kill cancer cells. This procedure, Pharisis (a cleansing of the blood), awakens the immune system.

Echinacea And Leukemia

Echinacea, a potent immune system stimulant, should not be administered to leukemia patients. Since echinacea works by causing white blood cells to multiply and since leukemia is a disease of overproliferation of white blood cells, it is contraindicated in these cases.

Buttermilk

Buttermilk soothes mouth ulcers caused by chemotherapy.

Four Reasons Cancer Patients Should Not Eat Animal Fat

1. Fat contains a high amount of calories, which stimulates the growth of cancer cells.
2. Fat is high in certain fatty acids, particularly linoleic acid, which stimulate the growth of cancer cells.
3. Fat changes the body's estrogen stores.
4. Animal fat contains the residue of the pesticides present in the animal's food.

Cancer-Forming Foods

All food plants produce their own chemicals as protection against attack by foreign substances. The substances in the following foods are chemicals in the food to protect these foods against insects. In a healthy body they are not a problem. However, when the immune system is compromised, they can be poisonous to the body. They can exacerbate existing cancers because, instead of protecting the body, the liver has to take time away from its normal activity of keeping the body cleansed to deactivate these chemicals.

The foods and their substances are:

- Black pepper — safferols
- Common American mushrooms — hydrazine
- Figs and parsley — dorleans
- Potato — alko alkaloids
- Coffee — quinones
- Chocolate and tea — theobromines
- Various herbs and honey — parizoladines and alkaloids
- Fava beans — visines
- Mustard — alio
- Alcohol — acid aldehydes
- Peanuts, nuts and corn — aflatoxins (mold)
- Beets, lettuce, spinach — nitrites

Invasion Of The Parasites

Tumors are benign before becoming cancerous. The tumor is invaded by a parasite, causing malignancy. Cancer patients are loaded with parasites. Kill the parasites with black walnut, wormwood and clover.

Cottage Cheese Helps Destroy Cancer Cells

Cottage cheese is high in sulfur-containing amino acids, which drive the necessary oxygen into the cells, completing the reaction that is necessary for the body to destroy cancer.

How Radiation Therapy Works

Radiation therapy works by destroying cancer cells. The cancer cells do not produce antioxidants, therefore they are vulnerable to the free radical activities triggered by the radiation. Normal cells have antioxidant defense and are less affected by the radiation although some damage does occur.

Unrecognizable

Cancer cells cover themselves with a sugarlike substance which makes it impossible for the immune system to recognize and destroy them. Therefore it is necessary to destroy this coating so the immune system can recognize the cancer cells. For the immune system to be effective, it must mark the cells with something it can recognize.

Cancer In The Future

By the year 2020 cancer will be eradicated because it will be detected at such an early stage that simply taking a pill or applying a laser-tipped needle to the tumor will cure it.

Cancer Cure

Injections of 714X, a camphor, nitrogen, ammonia combination, discovered by a Canadian biochemist, Dr. Gaston Naessens, stops the excretion of the hormone that blocks the immune system. Cancer treatment in the United States is designed to attack the cancer, disregarding any therapy to stimulate the immune system.

They Don't Want You To Get Well

High levels of DHEA, an adrenal hormone, can prevent cancer. This was discovered by a Temple University Professor whose grant was subsequently rescinded.

Dr. Kelley's Cancer Program

Dr. Kelley's cancer program consisting of pancreatic enzyme therapy should be used only 15 days at a time to prevent the patient from becoming too toxic. It is essential to use coffee enemas to rid the body of toxins.

Tumor Marker Testing

Following cancer surgery, chemotherapy is often recommended to destroy any other cancer cells that might be present in the body. Before starting this dangerous therapy, tumor marker testing should be performed to determine if there are still cancer cells present. The statement, "We got it all," should be proven by the following tumor marker tests:

- CEA — Shows cancer enzyme activity
- LASA — A liver test
- CA 15-3 — Breast cancer tumor marker
- AMAS — Shows activity of antibodies against cancer
- CA 125 — For uterine cancer
- CA 19-9 — For colon cancer

Natural Healing Treatments For Treating Cancer

1. Ukraine (an herb)
2. 714X — camphor, nitrogen, ammonia combination (self-administered injections)
3. Amagdylin (Laetrile)
4. Mistletoe (an herb)
5 Shark cartilage
6. Thymus extract
7. ESSIAC — herb combination of burdock root, rhubarb, slippery elm bark and sheep sorrel
8. Hoxey treatment (herbs)
9. Antioxidant supplements — Vitamins A, C, E, riboflavin (B^2), beta-carotene, pycnogenal and coenzyme Q-10.
10. Plant antioxidants — mushrooms (shiitake, maitake, reishi)
11. Green tea
12. Soy protein
13. Cat's claw (an herb)
14. Oxygenating therapies — ozone, DC4, hydrogen peroxide

Interferon

Interferon, used as an immune system stimulant for patients with cancer and hepatitis, has side effects of severe flu-like symptoms, aching and depression.

11 Childhood Afflictions

Stop Stuffing The Children

The number one cause of vomiting in young children is overfeeding.

Implants And Breast-Feeding

Breast-fed children whose mothers had silicone breast implants have shown abnormal movement in the esophagus. This leads to digestive problems.

Human Milk

Human milk contains 55 percent fat. Colostrum in this fat and in the protein contains immune factors to protect the child for the first few days of life. Also, borage oil, found only in mother's milk, and the herb, borage, carries essential fatty acids (gamma linolenic acid) also needed to protect the child from viruses, bacteria and pathogens.

Commercial Infant Formula

Commercial infant formula contains two of the most highly saturated fats, palm oil and coconut oil.

Substitute Baby Formula

Babies allergic to cow's milk and soy-based formulas can tolerate Nutramagin. Since there is less calcium in this formula, babies should be supplemented with two teaspoons of Neocalglucon at bedtime.

No Skim Milk For Baby

Children under the age of two should not drink skim milk because they need fat to help build the central nervous system.

Botulism Warning

Do not give babies under one year old honey. It could cause botulism.

Nutrients By Juicing

Children who do not like leafy green vegetables can get their nutrients if you juice the vegetables and mix them with a little fruit juice.

Highly Allergic Foods

Foods likely to cause an allergic response leading to ear infections in children are:

- Wheat .... 33 percent
- Eggs .... 25 percent
- Peanuts .... 20 percent
- Soy .... 17 percent
- Corn............. 15 percent
- Oranges .... 10 percent
- Tomatoes ..... 5 percent
- Chicken .... 5 percent
- Apples .... 4 percent

Febrile Seizures

To prevent fever-related seizures in children, do not lower body temperature too rapidly. A cold water bath, or alcohol applied to their bodies causes the body temperature to drop too rapidly and shocks the system. Instead, lower temperature by using room temperature water for a half-hour.

Ear Drainage Tubes Fail

Children with recurrent ear infections often have drainage tubes inserted. These tubes can act as a channel for bacteria to infiltrate the inner ear. In addition, when the tubes are removed, scar tissue forms, trapping the bacteria which damages the inner ear, and this can lead to tinnitus or Ménière's disease later in life.

Most children's ear problems are caused by allergies rather than infections.

True Cause Of Ear Infections

Recurrent ear infections in children show that the way they've been treated is not effective. The underlying cause of the infection is not being addressed. It is essential to see if an allergy to wheat, eggs, dairy, or citrus, or a sensitivity to sugar is present. A high percentage of ear infections disappear when these dietary concerns are addressed.

Failure Of Antibiotics

When a child is prescribed antibiotics for ear infections, and they constantly recur, it indicates that antibiotic therapy is not effective. A program of investigating food allergies should be started.

Natural Therapy For Ear Infections And Sore Throat

Children with ear infections and/or strep throat can be effectively treated by giving them 10 drops of echinacea in tea every hour. Apply garlic and mullein mixed with olive oil to the ear.

Lead Lowers IQ

In Northern California, the average IQ of children has been reduced by 4 to 8 points from the lead in the environment.

Effect Of PCB

Children born to mothers with high concentrations of PCB (polychlorinated byphenols), dioxin, DDT and/or other endocrine-disrupting chemicals in their bloodstream showed the following damaging effects:

- Small penis size
- Reduced muscle tone
- Abnormally weak reflexes
- Poor performance on tests requiring fine motor coordination

American children with so-called normal amounts of PCB in their bloodstream also show slight physical and emotional retardation.

Stop Poisoning Our Children

Fifteen percent of all American children have been poisoned by lead-based paint in their homes and by lead from gasoline. Lead poisoning has no physical symptoms (it's a totally silent disease). However it affects children mentally and their scholastic achievement is impaired.

Sudden Infant Death Syndrome

Babies should sleep on their sides for the first three months to prevent SIDS (Sudden Infant Death Syndrome).

Sleep Patterns

From birth to three months children do not produce melatonin (a hormone produced in the pineal gland during the night which activates normal sleep patterns). That may be why they do not have regular sleep cycles.

Prenatal Ultrasound

Animal studies have shown that ultrasound causes birth defects.

Forego Green Grass

Children whose yards have been sprayed with insecticides have a four times greater rate of cancer.

Perilous Vaccine

Pertussis (whooping cough) vaccine acts on the pancreas and sometimes causes it to overproduce insulin. This can cause low blood sugar in infants, leading to brain damage.

Don't Depend On Pertussis Shots

Pertussis vaccine is only 80 percent effective. One of every 5 children vaccinated will still contract whooping cough. Therefore the risks are far greater than the benefits.

Vaccine Safety Test

To test for an allergic reaction to a vaccine, place a drop of the solution under the child's tongue and check to see if the pulse rate increases.

Danger Of Vaccinations

One side effect of vaccines that is dangerous to children is the possibility of impairment to the nerve coverings. This could be a cause of multiple sclerosis.

Crib Death

Most crib deaths occur 36 hours following immunizations.

Seizures From DPT Shots

The pertussis portion of DPT vaccine causes high fevers ranging from 102 to 105 degrees in 50 percent of babies. High fevers can lead to seizures, paralysis, dyslexia and cerebral palsy, which occurs in 1 of 500 cases within 24 hours of the injection. The effect of the vaccine is cumulative and reactions increase in severity with each subsequent shot. In addition, medical text books state that any child who has seizures should not be given the pertussis portion of the vaccine. Parents of children who suffered from seizures within 24 hours of the shot, and refused to continue the series, were told by school officials that children would not be enrolled unless the series was completed. For more information on this topic, read *"A Shot In The Dark"* by Harris Coulter.

12 Cholesterol

French Phenomenon

Latest studies from France show that, in spite of a diet containing large amounts of butter and fat, the French have 63 percent less chance of having heart attacks than Americans. Their high consumption of wine is a contributing factor to this phenomena. The French also consume much less sugar than Americans and purchase fresh foods daily.

Normal Cholesterol Readings Meaningless

Eighty percent of heart attack victims have normal cholesterol readings.

Low Fat Diet Fails

When a doctor recommends a low fat diet for weight reduction or to lower cholesterol, the patient automatically starts eating higher amounts of carbohydrates. This diet ultimately leads to weight gain, higher cholesterol and higher triglycerides.

Low Cholesterol Diet Fails

A low cholesterol diet is a high carbohydrate diet. Since carbohydrates eventually convert to sugar, this type of diet can cause problems for diabetics and can also lead to weight gain.

Cholesterol-Lowering Drugs

Lowering cholesterol with drugs reduces the production of serotonin, a brain neurotransmitter needed to balance emotional hormones.

Fasting Lowers Cholesterol

Patients whose dangerously high cholesterol levels fail to respond to medication can greatly reduce these levels by fasting for four days under the supervision of a holistic physician. Be sure to drink enough water so you don't get dehydrated.

High Cholesterol Readings

High cholesterol readings without any mention of other coronary risk factors are meaningless.

Cholesterol And DDT

Exposure to DDT can raise HDL (good cholesterol). DDT is still being used in some foreign countries that supply us with food, including coffee grown in Brazil. This is just a point of interest and not something I recommend, as DDT has many harmful side effects.

Wine Raises Good Cholesterol

Wine with meals increases HDL by 10 percent.

Cholesterol Is Necessary

Cholesterol is not found in plants, only in animal food. Therefore, a strictly vegetarian diet does not contain cholesterol which is extremely necessary for a multitude of bodily functions. Without this very necessary sterol, many malfunctions can occur.

Cholesterol And Mental Health

Low cholesterol can cause depression severe enough to lead to suicide. The highest amount of cholesterol in the body is in the brain. Low cholesterol causes a reduction of the neurotransmitter, serotonin, which is one of the most important mood enhancers.

Shellfish Lowers Cholesterol

The type of cholesterol found in mollusks (clams, oysters, mussels) is a phytosterol which lowers the body's cholesterol. Caution — Be sure these shellfish come from unpolluted waters.

Medical Establishment Hype

The medical establishment states that everyone should be on the same diet, basically low fat and high carbohydrates. This is a generalization that does not apply to all people. All carbohydrates convert to sugar, and people with diabetes or low blood sugar (hypoglycemia) should be careful of their sugar intake. In addition, most carbohydrates cause more of a weight gain than animal-type foods.

The statement by the medical profession that high cholesterol foods are dangerous to your health is not true. They have the public convinced that all cholesterols are bad. However, without an adequate amount of cholesterol in our bodies, we would lose the ability to fend off disease.

When people are told something, such as cholesterol is bad for their health, they go to the other extreme and eliminate it entirely instead of just reducing the amount consumed. Eliminating animal-type food and eating large amounts of carbohydrates leads to elevated blood pressure, elevated blood sugar levels and weight gain.

Beans And Tofu

The type of protein derived from beans and tofu lowers cholesterol.

Oat Bran Overrated

Oat bran is not a panacea for lowering cholesterol. The main reason it works is that people eat it in place of bacon and eggs for breakfast.

Cholesterol Lowers Cholesterol

A Finnish study demonstrated that, for every milligram of cholesterol ingested, the body suppressed the manufacture of 2.2 mg in the body. Therefore the consumption of so-called cholesterol-high foods such as eggs, butter, cheese and meats actually causes the body to produce less cholesterol. These cholesterol-high foods are not what causes cholesterol levels in the blood to rise. Saturated fats are the culprits.

Balance

Your system is in balance if your cholesterol reading is 100 points higher than your triglyceride reading. A normal cholesterol reading should range from 180 to 220. With less than a hundred point difference, you may not be assimilating carbohydrates properly. If the difference is greater than 100 points, the system will not tolerate fats.

Medication And Longevity

Cholesterol-lowering medication lowers cholesterol levels but does not necessarily extend your lifespan.

Lifespan

People with cholesterol readings ranging from 200 to 225 have the longest lifespans.

National Phobia

Dietary cholesterol does not always convert to blood cholesterol. A study was performed on an 80-year-old man in England who ate 25 eggs a day for several years and had a cholesterol reading of 180. Cholesterol-lowering drugs have never been shown to extend life, only to lower cholesterol minimumly, and they have harmful side effects.

Cholesterol has become a national phobia even though there are many, much more important risk factors, such as:

- Excess iron
- Insufficient amounts of antioxidants (Vitamins C, E, beta-carotene and selenium)
- Magnesium deficiency
- Lack of essential fatty acids
- Stress
- Smoking
- Sedentary lifestyle

- High homocysteine levels
- Platelet aggregation (blood platelets become sticky and cause clotting)
- Diabetes

Low Levels Can Be Dangerous

People with cholesterol levels below 125 have a high incidence of cancer, accidental death and suicide. Low cholesterol affects you psychologically because brain cells contain high amounts of cholesterol.

Pycnogenol

Pycnogenol, found in grape seeds, is the component in wine that lowers cholesterol. Pycnogenol is a bioflavanoid that is also abundant in tea, onions, apples and pine bark.

Healthy Beverages

Bioflavanoids can be derived from wine and tea, especially green tea. This is one reason for the low incidence of cholesterol problems among French and Asian people.

Children Need Cholesterol

Cholesterol is an important building block for the central nervous system, especially in young children. Therefore, parents who are limiting their children's cholesterol intake because of the current cholesterol phobia are doing their children a grave injustice.

Lowering Triglycerides Lowers Cholesterol

Low HDL usually coexists with high triglycerides (circulating blood fats). Therefore, lowering triglycerides will raise HDL.

For every 100 points that triglyceride levels are lowered, cholesterol levels will fall by 20 points. Triglyceride levels can be lowered by eating fewer simple carbohydrates such as fruit, fruit juice, dried fruit and processed sugar products. In addition, fish oil, chromium picolinate and garlic help to lower triglyceride levels.

Daily Garlic

One clove of garlic daily can reduce cholesterol levels by 23 points.

Good Cholesterol

Chromium picolinate raises HDL (good cholesterol).

Margerine Spells F A T

Transfatty acids found in margarine and commercial baked goods raise cholesterol, even though the labels say no fat or low fat.

Why Cholesterol Is Necessary

Cholesterol is crucial for the manufacture of the critical hormones and nutrients Vitamin D, DHEA, estrogen, progesterone, testosterone and cortisone. Lowering cholesterol levels too much is injurious to optimal production of these hormones.

Check Your Thyroid

High cholesterol and high triglycerides can be caused by low thyroid function.

Better Eggs From Better-Fed Chickens

Chickens fed flaxseed produce eggs that contain less cholesterol. Those who consume two of these eggs daily increase their HDL levels and lower their triglycerides.

Complex Carbs May Be Dangerous

Diets using high complex carbohydrates to lower cholesterol levels also raise insulin levels, placing these dieters at an even greater risk of developing heart disease even though their cholesterol levels may be reduced.

Consider The Ratio

HDL readings should be taken into consideration before recommending cholesterol-reducing medication. Even with total readings in the 300 range, if the HDL is 75 or above, it is inappropriate to give medication. The risk factor ratio of 4 to 1 or less is not indicative of a heart problem and 300 to 75 is a 4 to 1 ratio (this is determined by dividing the total cholesterol by the HDL).

Lipoprotein "A"

Lipoprotein A should also be measured when your cholesterol it tested. Even with a normal cholesterol reading, if your Lipoprotein A is elevated, there is a 15 times greater risk of stroke. High levels are also seen in people who have heart attacks. Fibrinogen and homocysteine should also be measured since high readings are predictors of occluded arteries.

High Carb Diet Fails

A low fat, high carbohydrate diet lowers cholesterol for about four to five months. Then cholesterol slowly rises to a higher point than when the diet was begun.

Chromium Picolinate

Chromium picolinate, 200 mg three times a day raises HDL, the "good" cholesterol.

Two Eggs Daily

People who ate two eggs daily from chickens whose feed consisted of fish meal containing Omega 3, Iodine and Vitamin E, actually reduced their cholesterol levels.

Eggs & HDL

Eggs raise HDL (the good cholesterol).

Lower Cholesterol Does Not = Long Life

Three cholesterol studies, the Minnesota Coronary Society, the World Health Organization and the Helsinki Heart Study, all showed that lowering cholesterol did not lengthen life and had a very low effect on reducing heart attacks.

None of those whose cholesterol was lowered fared any better than the untreated group. And in fact, the treated group had a higher incidence (242 percent) of death from heart disease.

Transfatty Acids

Transfatty acids in margarine and certain baked goods clog the receptors on the cells. These receptors are responsible for taking in specific chemicals needed by the cell to regulate cholesterol levels.

Banned In Japan

Cholesterol-lowering drugs also lower Coenzyme Q-10 levels in the body. Because of this dangerous side effect, cholesterol-lowering medication has been banned in Japan. Coenzyme Q-10, a crucial substance which is manufactured in every cell of the body, is needed for:

- Strengthening the immune system
- Reducing high blood pressure
- Protecting the gums from periodontal disease
- Adequate heart muscle function

How To Lower Cholesterol Naturally

There are three ways to lower cholesterol naturally:

- Avoid transfatty acids
- Exercise
- Don't smoke (not because of the nicotine, because of the carbon monoxide)

The Value Of Cholesterol

Cholesterol is needed for the production of testosterone in the body. Most vegetarian diets lack cholesterol and, therefore, the production of necessary hormones is impaired.

Protect Your Arteries

Lipoprotein A is the material responsible for making LDL stick to the inside wall of the artery.

Lysine and Proline (amino acids derived from animal sources) form a teflon-like coating on the arterial wall, preventing the LDL from adhering to it.

Hibernating Bears

Cholesterol levels of hibernating bears range from 400 to 600, but they do not die from heart attacks. One reason is that animals manufacture their own Vitamin C, which is important for the production of collagen, the substance needed to keep the artery healthy.

What's More Dangerous Than Cholesterol?

Insulin is much more dangerous to the system than cholesterol. It will eventually destroy the nerve endings and arteries.

Don't Rely On Low Cholesterol

Patients who have heart disease and yet have low total cholesterol levels should have other possible causes, such as lipoprotein A levels and homocysteine levels, looked into. They should also be tested to see if their HDL (good cholesterol) levels are too low.

Medium Chain Triglycerides

Medium chain triglycerides lower cholesterol and enhance energy, and they are easy for the liver to metabolize and absorb. Known as MCT's, they are available in health food stores.

Don't Starve For The Test

Fasting for a cholesterol test is not necessary since the levels do not change when the stomach is empty.

Foiled By The FDA

Guar gum, a very effective cholesterol-lowering food supplement, was removed from the market by the FDA. This is another example of the FDA eliminating an effective natural treatment with full disregard for the health and well-being of the average American.

Good Cholesterol Lacking

It is very difficult to raise good cholesterol (HDL) if you are on a vegetarian diet. You need some animal protein for this process to happen.

Check The Ratio

Heart disease is rare if you have high HDL (good cholesterol) even if your total cholesterol levels are also high.

Futile Treatment

Cholesterol-lowering medication will not work if your HDL is high. With high HDL, it would be stupid to prescribe such medication since high HDL is a protective factor.

13 Dental

Dental Implants

Dental implants should be made of titanium, not nickel or stainless steel, which can cause an adverse reaction in the body and depress the immune system. Before any foreign material is used in the mouth, a material compatibility test should be performed. Fourteen percent of people react to gold, only one percent react to titanium. Mercury is the most toxic of all the heavy metals, and 52 percent of silver fillings consist of mercury.

Toxic Fillings

Silver fillings contain copper, which can exacerbate Wilson's Disease (a hereditary condition whereby the liver cannot properly metabolize copper). Copper accumulates in the liver and could lead to hepatitis. The term silver fillings (also called amalgam) is a misnomer. The material contains only 16 percent silver, and the rest is mercury and copper, highly toxic heavy metals which poison the system and depress the immune system.

Double Standard

EPA regulations prohibit dentists from disposing of mercury in the sewer system or in regular trash. It must be disposed of in a toxic waste site. They cannot let mercury come in contact with their skin. Yet this highly toxic mercury is used in amalgam fillings in the teeth.

Poison In Your Teeth

Mercury is more poisonous than arsenic. Silver fillings are 52 percent mercury.

Europe Bans Silver Fillings

Most European countries have banned silver amalgam fillings because they contain high amounts of mercury which depresses the immune system. However, in the United States, dentists are oblivious to this pertinent fact and still continue to use the material, with devastating results.

After Removing Silver Fillings

Individuals who have amalgam fillings removed should undergo chelation therapy immediately afterward to rid their body of the toxic effects of the mercury.

Fluoridation Fails

Europeans do not fluoridate their water supply, yet have fewer cavities than Americans.

Toxic Toothpaste

Most toothpaste contains 1500 parts per million of fluoride, and toxic levels are 4 parts per million.

Side Effect Of Novocaine

The adrenalin in novocaine can cause an increase in heart rate. Dentists should be aware of this when treating patients with heart disease.

Aid For Sensitive Teeth

Strontium chloride in toothpaste helps to reduce tooth sensitivity. It is a newly recognized and important constituent of bone.

Danger Of Root Canal

A dead tooth in the mouth can't defend itself against the bacteria that is trapped in its root, which eventually turns anaerobic and toxic to the body because it does not have a blood supply.

Swollen Glands

When no other cause can be found, chronic swollen glands in the neck may be due to an infected root canal.

Dental Procedure Shrinks Testicle

If a male under age 18 has a root canal performed on a front tooth, the testicle on that side may atrophy to about one-half normal size.

Low White Blood Count

A low white blood count can be due to an infection in a root canal.

Relieve Canker Sores

To relieve canker sores, eliminate citrus and nuts from the diet, and rinse the mouth with licorice tea three times daily. Do not swallow the tea. Suck on deglycyrrhizinated licorice lozenges.

Two For One

The panoramic X-ray taken by dentists to diagnose lower jaw problems also shows if plaque is present in the carotid arteries.

Toothless Seniors

One out of three people over 65 have lost all their teeth.

14 Diabetes And Hypoglycemia

Check Insulin Levels

When testing for diabetes or hypoglycemia, if a glucose tolerance test is performed without first ascertaining insulin levels, the test is meaningless. This is because, if the pancreas is still producing insulin, this patient is not a true diabetic.

Leg Ulcers

Patients with leg ulcers should keep the leg elevated in order to prevent the stagnation of blood which causes infection and inflammation. Use honey on the ulcers as a topical antibiotic.

Blood-Sugar-Lowering Medication

All blood-sugar-lowering medications increase the chance of developing a heart condition. With lower blood sugar readings, patients have a false sense of security and start to consume more carbohydrate-type foods. Eventually this increases their risk of having a heart attack 2 1/2 times because carbohydrates convert to sugar, causing higher production of insulin. Insulin is a growth hormone that destroys the material lining the arteries, including the coronary arteries, and this eventually leads to occlusion of these arteries and ultimately a heart attack.

Insulin Shots

Insulin shots should not be administered in the same area every time, or scarring will occur.

Insulin Increases Appetite

Diabetics on insulin therapy tend to gain weight because insulin acts directly on the brain as an appetite enhancer.

Too Much Insulin

If diabetics receive too much insulin (an atherogenic material which produces plaque), it will eventually lead to blocked arteries. Studies show that, if insulin is injected into arteries and monitored visually, plaque deposits can be seen forming inside the arteries.

The accumulation of too much insulin in the system causes destruction of DNA material in the cells lining the arteries. This is the beginning of the formation of plaque. In cases of adult-onset diabetes where insulin levels are not checked (C-Peptide Test), it is possible the patient is already producing an adequate amount of insulin, and giving extra insulin could be downright dangerous. These people can control their diabetes merely by cutting down on the amount of carbohydrate food they consume.

Beware Of Insulin

A side effect of insulin is cell leakage which can cause retinopathy, leading to blindness. Insulin induces the uptake of too much cholesterol into the cells. An overabundance of cholesterol in the cell causes eventual dysfunction. It also causes sodium retention by stimulating the sympathetic nervous system, thereby raising blood pressure. It can cause growth of cells in arteries, leading to atherosclerosis.

Vitamins Heal Damaged Nerves

Injections of Vitamins B^1, B^6 and B^{12} can restore the conductivity of damaged nerves in cases of diabetic neuropathy. Ointment containing extract of cayenne red pepper can be applied topically to the affected areas.

Dangers Of The Glucose Tolerance Test

A glucose tolerance test can be dangerous for some people. If the patient is hypoglycemic and the blood sugar falls to an extremely low level, seizures could occur. Patients with low normal blood sugar could also suffer from seizures after overindulging in sugar which causes their blood sugar to drop to dangerously low levels.

Silent Heart Attacks

Diabetics are prone to silent heart attacks. The nerve endings carrying transmission of pain to the brain are so dysfunctional from the diabetes that these diabetics don't feel any sensation in their chests from the blockage of the coronary vessel.

Long-Term Cortisone Therapy

Prolonged use of cortisone therapy can cause diabetes. Cortisone is only addressing the symptoms of disease. The patient must address and eradicate the cause of the condition in order to eliminate the necessity of taking cortisone.

Weight Distribution

Those people whose weight is concentrated in their midsection have high insulin levels which eventually leads to hypoglycemia. They should be on a high protein, low carbohydrate diet, which will help them lose weight.

Medication Backfires

Medication given for adult-onset diabetes lowers blood sugar so much that it causes an increase in appetite. This stimulates a craving for carbohydrates which in turn causes a rise in blood sugar, offsetting the purpose of the medication. Patients can get their blood sugar to a normal level by staying on a high protein, low carbohydrate diet and using supplements of chromium picolinate, zinc, biotin, vanaldyl sulfate, L-Alanine (an amino acid) and the herbs blueberry, juniper berries and goldenseal.

Beware Of Blood Pressure Medication

Blood pressure medication raises insulin levels which is dangerous for a diabetic. Lower your blood pressure naturally by dieting if overweight and by incorporating meditation and biofeedback into your daily routine. Useful supplements are Vitamin C and B^6, L-Taurine and the herbs garlic and Hawthorne berries.

Diabetes Damages Bones

Diabetes causes acidosis (high acid condition of the blood). In the body's attempt to buffer this high acidity, calcium is leached from the bones. The body has to be made more alkaline by including more vegetables and fruits in the diet and by decreasing the amount of grains, sugars and animal fats which are acid-producing.

Early Warning System

Diabetes is a systemic condition that may start to affect the nerves even before the condition is formally diagnosed. For example, numbness in the hands and feet may be an early indicator.

Insulin Can Be Deadly

Most of those with adult-onset diabetes actually have enough insulin. Instead of administering substances that would allow for more release of the body's own insulin, such as goldenseal, juniper berries, blueberry herbs, and glandular pancreas, far too many orthodox practitioners prescribe insulin which eventually leads to peripheral neuropathy, a condition leading to gangrene with eventual amputation, kidney disease and retinal disease. Most diabetics are deficient in chromium, zinc and magnesium and should be sure these are included in their vitamin/mineral supplements.

Retinal Bleeding

Shark cartilage is effective for retinal bleeding in diabetics. It controls the perfusion (overgrowth) of new blood vessels which can cause bleeding in the retina of the eye because the new vessels are not as strong as the original vessels.

Misdiagnosis Of A Sugar Problem

In a glucose tolerance test, the liquid sugar is made from corn syrup. Anyone allergic to corn could have a reaction to the liquid and this could be mistaken for a sugar problem.

The Natural Way Is Best

Diabetics have higher levels of free radical damage. Insulin promotes production of free radicals in the body. The benefits of synthetic insulin may be offset by its side effects. Therefore, a natural method of treating diabetes should be incorporated.

In cases of adult-onset diabetes, when a high blood sugar level is present and the patient is overweight, blood sugar levels can often be brought down to normal by simply eliminating carbohydrates and losing weight.

Vitamin C Lowers Insulin Requirements

Diabetics can lower insulin requirements by taking Vitamin C. For every 1000 mg of Vitamin C, insulin dosage can be decreased by two and a half units.

Blood Sugar Regulator

Progesterone helps regulate blood sugar.

Vitamin C Deficiency

Since the transport of Vitamin C to the cells is helped by insulin, many diabetics do not have enough Vitamin C in their cells. Therefore they may have a Vitamin C Deficiency in spite of what is considered an adequate intake of this vitamin in their diet. Non-insulin-dependent diabetics have also been shown to have low levels of plasma Vitamin C, as determined by a blood test called C-Peptide.

15 Diet And Weight Control

Viva La France

Latest studies from France show that in spite of a diet containing large amounts of butter and fat, the French have a 63 percent smaller chance of having heart attacks than Americans. Their high consumption of wine is a contributing factor to this phenomena. The French also consume much less sugar than Americans.

Deficiencies Of Pritikin Diet Plan

The Pritikin diet plan does not include the use of supplements, and the diet is deficient in essential fatty acids because of the lack of animal-type food. This deficiency could cause menstrual and menopausal problems, inflammation, thyroiditis and the exacerbation of autoimmune diseases such as arthritis, lupus and multiple sclerosis.

The Right Diet May Be Wrong For You

The medical establishment states that everyone should be on the same diet, basically low fat and high carbohydrates. This is a generalization that does not apply to all people. All carbohydrates convert to sugar, and people with diabetes or low blood sugar (hypoglycemia) should be careful of their sugar intake. In addition, most carbohydrates cause more of a weight gain than animal-type foods.

The statement by the orthodoxy that high cholesterol foods are dangerous to your health is not true. They have the public convinced that all cholesterols are bad. However, without an adequate amount of cholesterol in our bodies, we would lose the ability to fend off disease.

When people are told something such as cholesterol is bad for their health, they go to the extreme of eliminating it entirely instead of reducing the amount. Eliminating animal-type food and consuming large amounts of carbohydrates leads to elevated blood pressure, elevated blood sugar levels and weight gain.

Veggies Hamper Breathing

Anyone with COPD — chronic obstructive pulmonary diseases (emphysema, bronchitis and asthma) — should not follow a strict vegetarian diet. Vegetables, fruits and grains are carbohydrates, and when they break down in the body, an excessive amount of carbon dioxide is produced, which has to be eliminated through the already overtaxed lungs. Therefore, a diet containing more fat and protein from animal-type food that breaks down into nitrogen and a smaller amount of carbon dioxide is healthier for these people.

Vegetarian Diet Lacks Nutrients

A vegetarian diet, although healthy for some people, may not be the best diet for others due to the lack of such nutrients as Vitamin D, B^{12} and the eight essential amino acids which can be derived only from animal-type foods. Protein derived from plant-type food is assimilated differently in the body and does not supply the same type of nutrients that the eight essential amino acids from animal-type food do.

A Little Fat Won't Hurt

A low fat diet dries out the body causing the proliferation of ailments such as eczema, seborrhea, psoriasis, dry mouth and eyes and itchy skin.

Danger Of Carbohydrates

Carbohydrate consumption lowers the blood sugar of some people so much that they crave even more carbohydrates. These eventually turn into fat which is deposited in tissues and the lining of the arteries, causing blockage of the heart's blood vessels.

Reactionary Foods

Most diseases are the body's overreaction to certain foods. If the patient follows an elimination diet and the problem disappears, only to reappear when a specific food is reintroduced, this can tell you which food is the culprit. This is especially helpful in diseases such as asthma, colitis, eczema, seborrhea, psoriasis and Candida (yeast).

How Long Is Your Intestinal Tract?

The argument for vegetarianism is that humans have the long intestinal tract that is necessary for the digestion of fruits, vegetables and fibrous-type plant food. Actually, humans have an intermediate size digestive tract midway between those of ruminants and carnivores. Ruminants include cattle, bison, buffalo, deer, antelopes and giraffes who have multi stomachs and long intestines. Carnivores include lions, tigers, wolves and other meat-eating animals which have short intestines to quickly rid their bodies of the toxic side effects of the meat. Humans' intestinal tracts are between the two which means they can consume both plant and animal-type food.

More Misinformation

The public has been misinformed that high protein diets cause calcium loss. The loss is only temporary and it ceases after a few months.

Diet And The Immune System

A vegetarian diet does not stimulate the immune system. You need animal protein to stay healthy.

Sugar Is Worse Than Fat

The latest dietary advice from the medical orthodoxy is to limit fats to 20 to 30 percent of the daily diet. At the same time they advise you to consume large amounts of complex carbohydrates in the form of starches such as rice, grains, pasta and fruit. These carbohydrates convert to sugar which in turn becomes body fat, the same as if the person was consuming animal fat.

Fat Cells Poison Body

Another reason to maintain ideal weight is that toxins are stored in fat cells. This is generally overlooked when detoxifying the body. Most detoxification procedures address only the blood and colon and ignore the fat cells.

L-Carnitine

L-carnitine (necessary for good heart health) is not found in a vegetarian diet.

Starchy Vegetables Raise Triglycerides

A vegetarian diet causes a rise in triglycerides due to excessive consumption of carbohydrates. This can exacerbate diabetes or a heart condition.

Poisonous Body Fat

Toxins and chemicals are stored in body fat. The thinner you are, the fewer toxins you accumulate.

Rise In Calories

Although average Americans have reduced the amount of fat in their diet, caloric consumption has risen by 200 points.

Athletic Performance

Athletes performed better on a high fat diet than on a high carbohydrate diet. They had longer endurance.

Protein Does Not Cause Bone Loss

The statement that protein ingestion causes bone loss was based on short-term studies performed on people who went on high protein diets for weight loss. Due to the results of these studies, everyone curtailed protein intake. In actuality, bone loss balanced out and ceased after four to five months. Protein is necessary for the continuation of growth patterns in cells, bone, blood and muscle.

Dieting Releases Toxins

When body fat is reduced by dieting, the toxins and stored chemicals in the fat that are released can cause adverse reactions in the bloodstream. Most symptoms from this toxic poisoning are headaches, reduced attention span, anemia, elevated liver enzymes and vision disorders.

When dieting, it is important to eliminate these accumulated toxins by drinking eight to ten glasses of water daily, getting adequate exercise and taking high amounts of Vitamin C.

Muscles

For every pound of muscle developed, the metabolism is enhanced and the body burns 50 more calories.

Jump Start The Metabolism

When a person seeks medical advice to lose weight, the physician often orders a blood test to determine if their thyroid function is low (hypothyroidism). If the test shows that thyroid function is low, synthroid (thyroid replacement hormone) is prescribed. The logic here is to replace whatever is lacking, in this case T4 (the hormone thyroxine), which is produced in the thyroid gland.

If the patient still does not lose weight and tests show the thyroid's function is still low, the doctors increase the dosage. In many cases this is still ineffective because the T4 has to convert into T3 (active thyroid), and this process is not occurring. This conversion takes place in the liver and peripheral body cells. When thyroxine is ineffective, cytomel, which is *already* T3, should be given to jump start the metabolism. Cytomel should be given in a timed-release form twice daily in order not to overstimulate the person.

While many people think fasting will help them lose weight, fasting actually further lowers the metabolism of the T3 into the active hormone. Zinc and selenium can enhance the conversion of T4 into T3.

Fat Consumption Down — Weight Up

The average American weighed ten pounds more in 1994 than in 1984 even though fat consumption was down. This weight gain is due to increased consumption of carbohydrates.

Ethnic Foods

To maintain good health, the largest part of your diet should consist of what your forefathers ate. Ethnic foods (your own) are best for you.

Low Nutrient Foods

In one year the average American consumes the following quantities of low nutrient foods.

- 756 donuts
- 60 pounds of cake and cookies
- 23 gallons of ice cream
- 7 pounds of potato chips
- 22 pounds of candy
- 200 sticks of gum
- 365 servings of soda
- 90 pounds of fat
- 134 pounds of refined sugar

Fats Fuel Runners

Runners on a high fat diet showed a 20 percent advantage in performance compared to those who loaded up on carbohydrates, and a 30 percent advantage over those on a normal eating program.

Eliminating Toxins

Fasting is, without a doubt, one of the best ways to treat most ailments. During the process, all toxins are eventually eliminated from the body because the person is not ingesting any food. The toxins and poisons causing the illness are eliminated in the urine and eventually, through the capacity of the individual's immune system, the body will fully recover. In fact, the standard, orthodox method of treating disease with medication and surgery does nothing to eliminate the poisons that are causing the disease in the first place.

Animals fast when they get sick. Humans should do the same. Fasting allows the body to conserve energy. If a tumor is present, the body will devour it during a fast. When the body is in a fasting state, it utilizes its fat reservoirs, and when these are gone it will digest the tumor. Toxins will also be eliminated. Fasting applies only to food. It is essential to drink clear water and green vegetable juices to help flush out the toxins.

Downside Of A Vegetarian Diet

A vegetarian diet lacks the cholesterol needed for production of all hormones in the body. Cell membranes and the myelin sheath depend on cholesterol to protect nerves.

Vegetarians consume more nightshades than those on a well-balanced diet. Nightshades are poisonous plants that, when eaten by animals at times of famine, cause joint inflammation. Plants in the nightshade family flower at nighttime to avoid attracting animals. Nightshades include tomatoes, white potato, eggplant, bell peppers, tobacco and paprika.

- A vegetarian diet lacks the essential amino acids.
- It contains no Vitamin D.
- It contains no Vitamin B^{12}.
- It is low in zinc.

Fresh green vegetables bind with minerals, stopping their absorption into the system.

Phytates from uncooked grains and oxalates from uncooked greens bind certain essential minerals and block their absorption.

A vegetarian diet is too high in carbohydrates which convert into glucose and could be dangerous for diabetics and hypoglycemics.

A vegetarian diet raises tryglyceride levels because of its high glucose content.

Protein And Bone Loss

A high protein diet has been touted by the medical orthodoxy as a cause of bone loss. However, football players consume huge amounts of animal protein and do not have bone loss.

Medium Chain Triglycerides

Medium chain triglycerides (MCT's) are metabolized in the liver, as are carbohydrates, and are converted to energy. Any portion that is not used is stored as energy, unlike unused carbohydrates which are stored as fat.

Downside Of A Low Fat Diet

It causes dry skin.
It predisposes the individual to allergies.
It compromises the immune system.
It stunts the growth of children.

82 Percent Overweight

Only 18 percent of all Americans maintain their proper weight.

Fat Kids

One of every five American teenagers is overweight.

Testosterone And Weight

Many people with weight problems have low testosterone levels.

Fat Is Not The Culprit

Since 1975 the rate of obesity has gone up 30 percent. In 1975, 26 percent of the population was obese. Now it is 34 percent. According to medical reports, this is caused by an overabundance of fatty foods. Yet, the USDA (United States Department of Agriculture) statistics show that less fat is being consumed. Since 1975 people have been eating more fish and chicken and less meat, eggs and butter, and using skim milk rather than whole milk. In fact, the meat and dairy industries have to advertise for business. If people are eating less fat, how come the percentage of obesity has risen? The answer is that the weight gain is due to the increased consumption of carbohydrates.

Eating Late Causes Weight Gain

Consuming the same type of calories later in the day that you normally would have had earlier in the day will lead to weight gain.

Americans Are Too Fat

The foremost health problem in America is obesity. One third of the population weighs 20 percent more than they should.

Avoid Low Calorie Diets

Low calorie diets slow down metabolism, causing you to gain weight eventually, even though you are actually consuming fewer calories.

Beware Of Sugar

Misinformation to the American public has the average person believing they will lose weight and be healthier by eating low fat foods. Actually many low fat foods are loaded with sugar. For example, low fat frozen yogurt is overly sweet and people are using jelly instead of butter as a spread. Sugar turns into body fat causing weight gain.

Exercise Lessens Appetite

Exercising before eating is beneficial because it increases calorie burning. Exercise can actually decrease the appetite by producing more of the brain chemical responsible for feeling full.

Waist Fat

Weight gain in the waist area is associated with high cholesterol, high triglycerides, diabetes and heart attacks.

Acupuncture Reduces Appetite

Acupuncture for diet control works by activating the specific sensor points in the body that are responsible for cravings.

Lose Weight — Live Longer

Since toxins reside in fat tissue, losing weight does add to longevity.

Enhancing Metabolism

For every pound of muscle developed, the metabolism is enhanced and the body burns 50 more calories.

Less Stress — Less Weight

Stress causes weight gain by releasing cortisol which increases sugar in the blood that subsequently turns into fat.

Fool The Brain

Fructo-Olegio-Saccharide (F.O.S.) is not absorbed by the system and fools the brain into thinking the body is satiated, thereby decreasing the appetite.

Weight Loss Diets Fail

One-quarter to one-third of the adults in the United States are overweight. Thirty-four million Americans can be classified as obese. Most people on weight loss programs experience initial success (a 10 percent loss of body weight). However, the long-term track record of weight loss programs is abysmal. One-third to two-thirds of the weight is regained within one year, and nearly all weight is regained within five years.

Only one in 250 dieters lose weight *without* regaining it. Ninety percent of the clients are repeaters who go from one weight loss program to another. This is a $33 billion dollar business which has no regulatory supervision.

Raise Your Thermostat

Thermogenesis is the production of heat in the body to burn fat and sugar as energy. The amount burned is determined by the effectiveness of the brown adipose tissue (BAT). Ma Huang (ephedra) should be combined with white willow bark and caffeine (kola nut) and cayenne red pepper to assist the BAT to produce heat leading to weight loss. The caffeine mobilizes the unwanted fat into the bloodstream and transports it to the brown adipose tissue. Anyone sensitive to caffeine can use ginseng as a mobilizer. Synthetic estrogen decreases the effectiveness of the BAT and is the reason why women on estrogen replacement therapy tend to gain weight.

16 Digestion

Beware Of Antacids

People suffering from heartburn, indigestion, burping and hiccupping may be deficient in hydrochloric acid and pancreatic enzymes. Taking these nutrients could alleviate the problem. They can be obtained in most health food stores.

Antacids usually cause more of a problem because they further deplete the acidity that is needed. They also contain aluminum, a toxic heavy metal that has been linked to Alzheimer's Disease, and talc which is poisonous to the system when ingested.

Blood Type/Digestion Connection

People with type A blood (40 percent of the population) are usually low in the hydrochloric acid needed for proper digestion and should take this nutrient if they have a problem.

Sweets Cause Bloating

High sugar consumption delays the emptying of the stomach, causing overproliferation of acids that lead to heartburn, gas, hiccupping and indigestion.

Intestinal Absorbant Area

If the absorbant area of the intestines were to be spread out flat, the area would be larger than a football field.

Medications And Leaky Gut

Medications contribute to leaky gut syndrome (the gut does not absorb properly, allowing toxins to leak into the bloodstream). They also slow the liver's process of detoxification.

Alleviate Leaky Gut

Fructo-Olegio-Saccharide and L. Glutamine help alleviate leaky gut and improve digestion. They also aid intestinal integrity and stimulate friendly bacteria.

Fluttering

Heartburn and gas can trigger heart palpitations.

Spice Up Your Life

If you suffer from such digestive problems as heartburn, gas and indigestion, you can improve your condition by eating spicy foods which stimulate rapid emptying of the stomach and higher acid levels.

Change Your Oil

Transfatty acids destroy the digestive process. Synthetically produced oils disrupt the natural enzymatic functions needed for the digestive process. Transfatty acids are found in margarine, hydrogenated oils and commercially baked products. Transfatty acids are produced because hydrogen is put into polyunsaturated oils such as sunflower, soy, corn and safflower when they are used in commercial products. Adding the hydrogen insures a longer shelf life because it eliminates oxygen which causes rancidity.

Polyunsaturated oils will become rancid quickly unless they are refrigerated. They also have a low flame point when used for cooking and food will burn. If using these oils, buy them in small quantities, don't cook with them and store them in the refrigerator.

For cooking and salad dressings, to eliminate the chance for oxidation and rancidity, use monounsaturated oils such as extra virgin olive oil, peanut oil, walnut oil, almond oil and sesame oil.

Transfatty acids have the following harmful effects. They:

- Double the risk of a heart attack.
- Interfere with a pregnancy.
- Cause low birth weight.

- Lower the quality of breast milk.
- Interfere with insulin function.
- Cause platelet aggregation.
- Interfere with liver detoxification.
- Change fat cell metabolism.

Wasting Disease

Patients with pancreatitis, an inflammatory condition of the pancreas causing lower production of pancreatic enzymes, should take pancreatin (a health food store product) to aid the digestive process. Otherwise, they will not properly metabolize food and may develop malnutrition severe enough to cause death. This is similar to the effect of pancreatic cancer on the body.

17 Epilepsy

Glucose Tolerance Test Dangerous To Epileptics

Epileptics should be wary of taking a glucose tolerance test because, if their blood sugar is reduced to a low enough degree, a seizure could occur.

IQ Lowered By Medication

Medications used to treat epilepsy have a tendency to lower the patient's IQ.

Supplements For Epilepsy

People with epilepsy may be helped by the following supplements: Vitamin B^6, Vitamin E, folic acid, manganese, taurine and zinc. These natural nutrients may be so effective that, eventually, anti-seizure medication will be unnecessary.

Don't Drink The Water

Tapeworm cysts were found in the Milwaukee water supply and caused seizures in some individuals.

Fat Stymies Epilepsy

A high fat diet is effective for treating epilepsy. It creates ketones which are fuel for the brain, and also alleviates the highs and lows from carbohydrates which are the cause of low blood sugar.

18 Eye Conditions

Eyes Diagnose Iron Deficiency

If the whites of your eyes have a blue tint, it could be a signal that you are deficient in iron.

Glaucoma Test

Drinking too much water before a glaucoma test can increase eye pressure and give a false positive reading.

Normal Eye Pressure

Even though eye pressure is normal, you could still have glaucoma.

Types Of Glaucoma

Not all people with high eye pressure develop glaucoma. The two types of glaucoma are:

- Closed angle, also known as fixed angle. This kind requires surgery.
- Open angle glaucoma, the more common type, means there is adequate circulation of fluid in the eye, but in time the circulation diminishes.

Effective Natural Glaucoma Remedy

Glaucoma is a circulatory disease. A combination of exercise along with 2 mg of Vitamin B^{12} daily is more effective in lowering the pressure than eye drops.

Eskimo Diet

Eskimos don't get glaucoma due to the high fat content of their diet.

Marijuana Works Wonders For Glaucoma

Marijuana and melatonin each lower intraocular pressure. Although marijuana is more effective, it can be difficult to obtain since it is classified as an illegal substance.

Use Preservative-Free Eye Drops

Preservatives in artificial tears can damage the cornea. If dry eyes are such a problem that moisterizing drops have to be used more than four times daily, be sure to use those without preservatives.

Contact Lenses

Contact lenses can cause corneal ulcers.

Radial Keratotomy

Radial keratotomy (a surgical procedure to alleviate nearsightedness) flattens the cornea, weakening the integrity of the eye. If trauma occurs in anyone who has undergone this procedure, their vision could be severely impaired.

Artificial Sweetener

Cloudy or blurred vision can be caused by an allergic reaction to aspartane, an artificial sweetener. People who have this happen are often unduly concerned that they may be developing cataracts, when they're not.

Warning To Myopics

Nearsighted people have a higher incidence of retinal detachment. Strengthen the retina by taking the following supplements: Vitamin A, B^2 (riboflavin), bioflavanoids, shark cartilage to stop bleeding, selenium and glutathione. It is also important to protect the eyes from UVA and UVB radiation by wearing proper sunglasses. Wear protective goggles when working in situations where the eyes could be injured. Avoid contact sports that might cause eye injuries.

Eye Color Significant

Individuals with light eyes are more susceptible to sun damage to the retina, so they should be sure to protect their eyes when out in the sunlight.

Detached Retina

Vitamin B^3 is useful as an additional treatment for detached retina.

Shark Cartilage Controls Bleeding Retina

Orthodox practitioners treat retinal neuropathy with laser therapy which is akin to putting a bandaid on the eye. This condition can be treated effectively with shark cartilage which stops the progression of bleeding in the retina. Use 20 grams daily. (Shark cartilage is usually available in 750 mg capsules. Use 26 of these daily.)

No Cause For Alarm

If the whites of the eyes appear bloody, but do not affect vision, they should clear up without treatment and not cause problems.

Eye Floaters

Myopic people tend to have more eye floaters than the average person.

The Cataract/Prednisone Connection

Long-term use of prednisone can cause cataracts.

Contacts And Cataracts

Contact lenses starve the cornea's tissue of oxygen and can eventually lead to cataracts.

Dangerous Accelerator

Macular degeneration is accelerated 20 times faster in people who have had cataract surgery.

Chalazions

Chalazions on the eyelid may be due to B^2 (riboflavin) deficiency. If you take extra B^2 with your B-complex, it could help alleviate the problem.

Eye Tics

If standard procedures for eye tics fail, try acupuncture which can often help.

Aspirin Damages Retina

Those with heart conditions, who also suffer from retinal bleeding caused by diabetic neuropathy, should not take aspirin or other blood thinners. If their blood is thinned too much, it could increase the retinal bleeding and could eventually lead to total blindness.

Taurine Treats Retina

The amino acid, taurine, is useful for treating problems of the retina where leakage occurs, either from injury or diabetic retinopathy.

Retinitis Pigmentosa

The orthodoxy offers no viable treatment for retinitis pigmentosa. However, excellent results have been reported among patients who increase their intake of Vitamin A from fish liver oil to 100,000 units daily. Important note: Vitamin A in such high amounts could be toxic to the liver. Patients should be monitored by periodic blood tests.

Contact Lens Warning

Acamphometra is a bacteria that can cause devastating corneal infections and result in severe pain and visual loss, possibly ending in the need for a corneal transplant. Eighty-five percent of the people with this condition wear contact lenses. To avoid this infection, use an effective disinfectant such as hydrogen peroxide on the lenses.

19 Female Conditions

Breasts

Exercise Affects Breast Milk

Nursing mothers who do aerobic exercises often find their babies dislike the taste of their milk. Exercise increases the production of lactic acid, giving the milk a sour taste.

Breast Implants

Saline-filled breast implants have a silicone covering that can be dangerous to the immune system.

Advantages Of Breast-Feeding For Babies

It enhances the immune system.

It is less colic. The baby does not swallow as much air since the breast is a better delivery system than a bottle, and babies are usually in a more upright position when breast-feeding.

Advantages Of Breast-Feeding For Mothers

There is a decreased chance of breast cancer. The number of hormonal cycles with fluctuating estrogens is reduced. Women who breast-feed have a 20 percent less chance of getting breast cancer before menopause.

Hormones released while nursing create a calmer, more responsive mother.

Nursing mothers have less postpartum depression.

Women who breast-feed lose weight around their hips faster. Note: Blessed thistle (an herb) aids in milk production.

Prolactin, Nursing And Infertility

Infertility could be due to a high prolactin level. Vitamin B^6 will block prolactin. Since prolactin is the hormone responsible for production of breast milk, nursing mothers should limit their intake of B^6.

Garlic

Nursing mothers who consume garlic often find their babies crave their milk.

B^6 — The Good And The Bad

Nursing mothers should not take Vitamin B^6 as it suppresses production of prolactin from the pituitary gland.

Conversely, if nipples leak, it is an indication of the overproduction of prolactin and B^6 can be used to regulate it.

Prolactin released during breast-feeding helps a woman relax.

Cystic Breasts

Hypothyroidism may cause cystic breasts. Iodine enhances thyroid activity. Sea kelp is an excellent source of iodine.

Calcifications In The Breast

Calcifications in the breast could be the result of previous fibrocystic breast disease and are not always necessarily indicative of cancer.

Protection From Mammography Radiation

For protection from exposure to radiation from a mammogram, rub Vitamin E oil into the breasts for three days prior to the study and take 800 I.U. of Vitamin E orally for the weeks prior to and following the proocedure.

Toxic Atmosphere

Our toxic atmosphere is one reason for the increase in the number of breast cancer cases. Chemicals get stored in fat tissue, and the breast contains the most fatty tissue in a woman's body.

USA Bad For Breasts

For every four women who die from breast cancer in China, 26 die in the United States.

Abortion And Breast Cancer

Abortion can increase breast cancer risk by 50 percent.

Smoking And Breast Cancer

Smoking can increase breast cancer risk 3000 times.

Contraceptive Pills

Drug companies state that contraceptive pills are safer today than when they were first used 30 years ago. It would be interesting to know if studies have been made on women who took the pill 30 years ago to see what their rates of breast cancer are.

Livestock Feed Affects Women

The breast cancer rate in Israel decreased by 30 percent from 1978 to 1988. During that time, they discontinued feeding pesticides and herbicides to livestock.

Cabbage Breast Wrap

If your breasts feel painful, try soothing them by inserting three green cabbage leaves in your bra when you go to bed at night.

Breast Cancer Prevention

One way to prevent breast cancer is to lower overactive estrogen levels by exercising.

Advantage Of Small Breasts

Certain body types demand extra vigilance. For example, women with large breasts have higher levels of breast cancer.

Tamoxifen—Unnatural Biological Therapy

If the latest studies of Tamoxifen show it is successful in the treatment of breast cancer, it will be prescribed as a preventive for the disease. This medication causes cessation or slowdown of the ovary's hormonal output which is an unnatural biological process and can lead to ill effects many years later.

Estrogen Blockers

Soy products work like Tamoxifen to block estrogen receptors on the breast. These products have no side effects.

Screening Mammograms

Mammograms on premenstrual women are not accurate due to the composition of the tissue in a young breast, which cannot be properly visualized because of its density.

Mammograms only show a mass. You can't see inside the mass with a mammogram. An ultrasound lets you see *inside* the mass to determine if it is a fluid-filled sac, which would only be a cyst, instead of a tumor, which is solid.

Screaming Mammograms

Overcompression of the breast during mammography can exacerbate an existing unknown cancer. Although some compression is necessary for a clear picture, be sure the technologist is not overdoing it.

High Cost Of Cleavage

Bras can harm the breasts. If they are too tight and consist of synthetic material, they can interrupt proper lymph drainage, possibly precipitating the eventual onset of cancer.

Increase In Cystic Breast Disease

In 1928, the incidence of cystic breast disease was three percent. By 1978 it had increased to 89 percent. One cause is the effect of xeno estrogens in our polluted atmosphere. Xeno estrogens are estrogens caused by combinations of harmful pollutants.

MENSTRUATION

Abnormal Menstrual Bleeding

Vitamin A is useful for abnormal menstrual bleeding. 50,000 I.U. can be taken daily until symptoms disappear.

Light And Menstruation

Blind women have abnormal menstrual cycles because light does not activate their pineal glands properly.

Ultra-Thin Women

Women whose body fat is 10 percent or less may not menstruate.

Anxiety And Depression In PMS

PMS accompanied by anxiety is usually caused by high estrogen and low progesterone. PMS accompanied by depression is usually caused by high progesterone and low estrogen.

Estrogen/Progesterone Ratio

Anxiety due to PMS may be an imbalance in the estrogen/progesterone ratio and can be alleviated by raising progesterone. 200 I.U. of Vitamin E and applications of Progest cream increase progesterone.

High Fiber For PMS

High fiber is useful for women who suffer from PMS since it absorbs excess estrogen.

PMS Barometer

Severe PMS can be an indicator of future menopausal problems.

Women And Heart Conditions

Menstrual periods protect women from heart conditions by naturally keeping iron levels down and blood thin.

Low Iron Levels

Vegetarians have low iron levels which is beneficial in older people with heart problems and arthritis. However, low iron levels can cause problems in premenopausal woman who are still menstruating.

Heavy Uterine Bleeding

Vitamin A can slow down heavy uterine bleeding.

Iron Controls Uterine Bleeding

Uterine bleeding is diminished by iron which thickens blood.

Overproduction Of Prolactin

A tumor on the pituitary gland can cause overproduction of prolactin, which can cause a woman to miss her period.

PMS / Menopause Connection

Women who suffer from PMS have higher rates of menopausal symptoms.

CONTRACEPTION

Birth Control Pills Deplete Essential Nutrients

Birth control pills diminish Vitamin B^6 and folic acid. Women using this method of birth control should supplement their diet with these nutrients.

Libido Lessened By Pill

Contraceptive pills block testosterone levels in women, decreasing their sex drive.

Condoms

Women may be allergic to latex condoms. Condoms lubricated with a spermacide can cause a bacterial infection. Lambskin condoms are not as effective as latex for prevention of sexually transmitted diseases.

Antibiotics Can Make You Pregnant

Antibiotics can render birth control pills ineffective. They speed up the metabolism of the contraceptive through the liver, reducing its effect. Women on birth control pills should use barrier methods of birth control while on antibiotic therapy.

Ineffective Contraception Method

Coitus interruptus (stopping intercourse before the male ejaculates) is not an effective means of contraception. The amount of semen produced before orgasm can be sufficient to cause a pregnancy.

Effectiveness Of Birth Control Methods

- Pill .... 93 percent effective
- Condoms .... 84.2 percent effective
- Diaphragm .... 78 percent effective
- Spermacides .... 69.8 percent effective

Diaphragms

Diaphragms can cause urinary tract infections in women.

INFERTILITY

Unripe Eggs

A cause of infertility could be polycystic ovarian disease, a condition where the ovary produces many eggs, but none of them ripen.

Acupuncture Aids Fertilization

In cases of infertility, when standard procedures fail, acupuncture is often effective.

Sperm Allergy

An allergy to her partner's sperm may be the cause of a woman's infertility. This can be overcome by having the woman build up her immune system by taking high doses of antioxidants, eating chemical-free organic foods, drinking distilled water, getting proper exercise and lowering her stress level.

Main Factors Preventing Pregnancy

1. Low or inadequate male sperm.
2. Anovulation — The egg is not released from the ovary into the fallopian tube.
3. Tubal factors — The egg may be impeded in its travel through the fallopian tube due to scarring from pelvic inflammatory disease (PID).
4. Cervical mucous may be too thick and may prevent the sperm from reaching the egg.
5. Low progesterone levels.

Adrenals And Infertility

If the adrenal glands produce too much testosterone and DHEA (male hormones), a female could become infertile and develop male characteristics. In these cases, low doses of hydrocortisone help balance adrenal function. Hyperactivity of the thyroid should also be investigated in this condition since a hyperactive thyroid causes the adrenals to malfunction.

PREGNANCY

Environment A Cause Of Miscarriages

Miscarriages are due to a luteal phase failure in the menstrual cycle. The egg and sperm form an embryo, but it does not develop because of a lack of progesterone. This is due to petrochemical contamination in the environment. These petrochemicals serve as very potent estrogenics, causing the imbalance of progesterone which then totally dominates the menstrual cycle.

Prevent Miscarriages

Fish oil is helpful in preventing miscarriages. Eskimos' pregnancies usually last 10 months. Most of their diet consists of fish.

Protect Your Baby—Deficiency In Folate

Pregnant women who take 800 mcg. of folic acid daily have a better chance of preventing neural tube defects such as spina bifida and central nervous system diseases in their infants. Latest studies show that a deficiency in folate during pregnancy can cause these defects.

Ease Nausea Of Pregnancy

Vitamin B^6 and ginseng will alleviate the nausea of pregnancy. Acupuncture is also effective.

Morning Sickness

Pregnant women have an enhanced sense of smell due to the extra estrogen in their systems. This is often the cause of morning sickness. Estrogen also enhances vision and a sensitivity to noise. To relieve morning sickness, suck on a lemon.

Cause Of Nausea In Pregnancy

Beta HCG, a female hormone produced in pregnancy and needed for growth of the fetus, is what causes nausea.

Joy Of The Second Trimester

The euphoria women feel during the second trimester of pregnancy is due to the large amount of progesterone released at this time. Progesterone also protects women from cancer.

Kitty Litter Dangerous

Pregnant women should not handle soiled kitty litter as it can cause toxic plasmosis, a blood disease detrimental to the fetus.

Fewer Miscarriages At North Pole

Fish oil with borage seed oil is beneficial to women to help prevent miscarriages. Eskimos, whose diet consists mainly of fatty fish, have low rates of miscarriages.

Nitro Patch's Extra Benefit

The nitroglycerine patch can slow down the dilation of the cervix and help prevent premature birth, allowing the pregnancy to continue and the fetus to grow.

Birth Centers

The cost of childbirth in a birth center is one-third that in a hospital. The caesarean rate in birth centers is one-half that of hospitals.

Mother's Anesthesia Affects Newborn's Brain Cells

The offspring of mothers who received large amounts of anesthesia during the birthing process have a higher likelihood of developing addictive-type personalities.

Anesthesia can slow labor and have negative effects on the fetus.

Ultrasound Studies Affect Fetus

Studies show that when pregnant women undergo multiple ultrasound studies, their children develop more allergies and illness.

Epidural Anesthesia Dangerous

Epidural anesthesia given during childbirth to alleviate pain can slow labor and have negative effects on the fetus.

Caesarian Sections And Hernias

Caesarian sections often lead to hernias because the surgery weakens the abdominal wall.

Legal Climate Causes Increase In Caesarians

Many obstetrician/gynecologists no longer deliver babies because of the threat of malpractice. The legal climate forces them to perform caesarians to protect themselves from lawsuits. The United States has the highest percent of caesarian sections in the world.

Post-Pregnancy Weight Gain

The average woman gains six pounds per pregnancy which she never loses.

Post-Pregnancy Hormone Levels

The reduction in high levels of hormones following a pregnancy is similar in effect to menopause. Women have to rebuild their levels of pre-pregnancy hormones by taking Change of Life Herbal Formula, folic acid, boron, Vitamin E, the herbs false unicorn and blessed thistle and using Progest cream.

Pregnancy Quells Autoimmune Disease

Pregnancy can cool down an overactive immune system (autoimmune disease) because the immune system becomes depressed due to the allergic reaction of the body to the fetus.

Postpartum Depression

Postpartum depression could possibly be due to low thyroid function or low progesterone levels.

Is It Depression Or Sleep Deprivation?

Postpartum depression is more likely caused by sleep deprivation than by a psychological reason. Mothers getting up several times a night are not getting adequate rest. Sleep deprivation is a form of torture used to interrogate political prisoners. Menopausal women whose sleep is disturbed with hot flashes also may display symptoms of depression.

MENOPAUSE

Periods May Be More Frequent When Approaching Menopause

The time between menstrual periods often gets shorter rather than longer when women enter menopause. Many women are unduly alarmed since they believe it logical for their periods to be further apart at this time of life.

Natural Estrogen Replacement

Estrogen produced by herbal remedies is different from that produced biologically and/or medically prescribed, and it does not act as a cancer enhancer.

Herbs for estrogen enhancement include ginseng, wild Mexican yams, black cohash, licorice root and sarsaparilla.

Artificial Estrogen Dangerous

Prescribed artificial estrogen does not have the same molecular configuration as a natural molecule of estrogen and may cause cancer. It is not true human estrogen, but is derived from *pre*gnant *mar*e ur*in*e, hence its name Premarin.

Estrogen And Weight Gain

Estrogen causes weight gain. This is the reason the hormone is given to animals that are used for human consumption.

Synthetic Estrogen And Gallbladder Surgery

Latest studies show a 50 percent increase in gallbladder surgery in postmenopausal women who use estrogen replacement therapy.

Sources Of Natural Estrogen

Ginseng, licorice and soy products are good sources of natural estrogen.

A Problem Of Progesterone

Progesterone, often administered with estrogen to prevent uterine cancer, can cause high blood pressure and headaches.

Exercise / Estrogen Connection

Women who exercise have a lower incidence of cancer due to the reduction of excess estrogen. Exercise regulates estrogen production.

Estrogen Stimulator

Vitamin E does not create estrogen in menopausal women, but it assists in the secretion of the hormone from the adrenal glands and muscle and fat tissue to the ovaries where it is needed. Herbs that assist in this process are black cohash, licorice root, ginseng and sarsaparilla.

Ovaries

The ovaries always produce some hormones even after menopause or removal of the uterus.

Low Progesterone

High estrogen levels accompanied with low progesterone levels cause the receptor sites in female organs to be inundated with too much estrogen, bringing about a dysfunction in the cells leading to the possibility of cancer. Low progesterone can occur when the adrenal glands have to overproduce adrenalin to cope with a high stress level when there are deficiencies of other nutrients. Since progesterone is an alternate stress hormone, a woman under stress will deplete her levels, thereby raising the estrogen/progesterone ratio. Low progesterone levels may cause PMS. Eventually, women who suffer from PMS also have problems with menopause.

Early Surgical Menopause

If the uterus is removed and the ovaries are left intact, fifty percent of the blood supply to the ovaries is diminished, precipitating menopause at an earlier age.

Natural Estrogens

Two natural estrogens, Estriol and Estrace, can be prescribed instead of the synthetic type. This eliminates the possibility of contracting female type cancers.

Benefits Of Progesterone

Most female problems are due to an imbalance of hormones—too much estrogen and not enough progesterone. Since progesterone is formed from cholesterol, the current mania to lower cholesterol is doing women an injustice. It is progesterone, not estrogen, that protects against the demineralization of bone leading to osteoporosis. Progesterone is also a vasorelaxant which eases menstrual cramps. Furthermore, it acts as a mood elevator.

Magnesium Aids Menopausal Symptoms

Magnesium is effective to decrease hot flashes and night sweats in menopause.

Cause Of Weight Gain In Menopause

Most women entering menopause have a tendency to gain weight because the lowered progesterone production causes the thyroid to reduce its output of thyroxine. This causes hypothyroidism leading to weight gain.

Thyroid levels can be raised by taking synthroid, which must be prescribed by a medical doctor, utilizing a weight loss program of high protein, low carbohydrates and using fat-burning type supplements such as ephedra (do not use ephedra if you are diabetic or have high blood pressure) with cayenne red pepper, white willow bark and kola nut which transport the fat so thermogenesis will be activated. Additional supplements for weight loss include L-Carnitine, chromium picolinate and soluble fiber such as pectin and psyllium seed. You should also do aerobic exercises.

Low Body Fat

Slender women with low body fat enter menopause with more symptoms than women with high body fat. The reason is that estrogen is stored in adipose (fat) tissue.

Vegetarian Diet

Women on vegetarian diets produce less estrogen than those who consume a high amount of animal-type food.

Downplaying Progesterone

At menopause there is a greater drop in progesterone than estrogen. Yet the orthodoxy overstresses the need for estrogen replacement. Estrogen replacement therapy slows bone loss. It does not rebuild bone. Progesterone rebuilds bone.

When a woman has had a hysterectomy, she is told progesterone is not necessary. But, in fact, progesterone is as important, or more so, than estrogen.

Natural progesterone (Progest cream) that has no side effects can be obtained in health food stores. It is made from Mexican wild yams. Cabbage also helps produce progesterone.

Other Body Sources Of Estrogen

In addition to the ovaries, estrogen is also produced in the liver, body fat, hair follicles, the pineal gland and the adrenals.

Night Sweats

Night sweats associated with menopause can mean food allergies are present. They may be due to a depressed immune system associated with a decrease in natural estrogen.

Exercise

Exercise raises natural estrogen in menopausal women.

Provera Protects Uterus

The reason for taking Provera (a form of progesterone) with estrogen replacement therapy is that when a woman takes estrogen and does not menstruate, tissue is built up in the uterus. If this tissue is not shed, it could cause cancer. Provera aids in the sloughing off of this tissue. If some bleeding does not occur when taking Provera, the dose is too low.

Cabbage Is A Girl's Best Friend

Indoles in the cabbage family deactivate harmful estrogen.

Fiber And Estrogen

A high fiber diet moderates estrogen production. It lowers estrogen levels by transporting the hormone out of the body.

Overactive Natural Estrogens

Phytoestrogens in soy products and cruciferous vegetables (cabbage family) block the harmful effects of overactive natural estrogens in the body. These estrogens may cause or exacerbate fibroid tumors, cystic breasts and endometriosis.

Killer Cell Activator

Natural killer cells diminish in numbers and activity as women approach menopause. To enhance natural killer cells at this time, you should take high amounts of antioxidants, including pycnogenal (grape seed extract).

Clinical Definition

The clinical definition of menopause is the cessation of menstrual periods for three years.

Depression

Women are no more likely to be depressed during their menopausal years than at other times in their lives. The highest rate of depression among women is for those in the 20 to 30 year age group who are at home with young children.

Some Menopausal Statistics

- 25 percent of women have no symptoms.
- 50 percent have moderate symptoms.
- 25 percent have severe symptoms.

Misconceptions

- Menopause is a deficiency disease.
- Menopause is a condition that ages women overnight.
- At menopause all women lose sexual desire.
- Hot flashes are all in the mind.
- Depression is a part of menopause.

Cause Of Hot Flashes

Hot flashes are not in the mind, but they are in the head. When the hypothalamus is estrogen-deprived, it sends out the wrong signal to the body, telling it to react as if the room were too hot.

REM Sleep Disturbed

REM or Rapid Eye Movement sleep is disturbed by hot flashes. This is one cause of depression and mood swings because anyone deprived of sleep becomes crabby. Sleep deprivation is a form of torture.

Medications And Dry Vagina

Antidepressants, blood pressure and heart medications are known to cause dry mouth, but they also dry out all mucous membranes, including the tissue lining the vagina and urinary tract making these areas more susceptible to infection.

OSTEOPOROSIS

Protein Robs Bones

Less bone loss will occur in patients with osteoporosis who adhere to a modified vegetarian diet rather than one containing large amounts of protein.

Calcium Carbonate Constipates

Tums™ have been touted as a good source of calcium. However, they contain the type of calcium (carbonate) which is difficult for the body to absorb, especially in older people with diminished digestive systems. Calcium carbonate can also cause severe constipation.

Chinese Prove Milk Not A Panacea

Even though the Chinese hardly consume any milk or other dairy products, they have very low levels of osteoporosis. This refutes the orthodox dogma that one must drink milk in order to have strong bones.

Overlooked Cause Of Osteoporosis

Allergies, diabetes and stress make the body acidic and cause calcium to be withdrawn from the bones to buffer this acidic state. Leaching calcium this way will eventually lead to osteoporosis.

Building New Bone

Estrogen can prevent osteoporosis. It protects the body against bone loss by aiding the thyroid and parathyroid glands in their regulation of calcium in and out of the blood and bones. Estrogen does not build new bone. That is a metabolic process derived from the chemical activity of calcium, magnesium, silica, boron, manganese and Vitamin C. Calcium alone cannot build new bone.

Progest Cream

The application of Progest cream, an extract of wild yams containing progesterone, will decrease the likelihood of osteoporosis in women. Topical progesterone (Progest cream) enhances bone density.

Avoid Drinking Soda

Phosphoric acid binds up calcium and prevents it from being utilized by the body. The largest concentration of phosphoric acid is found in carbonated soft drinks. Women with a tendency toward osteoporosis should avoid drinking soda.

Chlorine Depletes Calcium

Chlorine in tap water carries calcium out of the body. Women prone to osteoporosis should drink filtered water.

Hormones Fail When Women Need Them Most

Latest studies show that hormone replacement therapy has to be taken for seven years to prevent bone thinning. Then its protective factors extend only to the 60th and 70th decade, not to ages 80 and 90 when most fractures and debilitating spinal compressions occur.

Magnesium And Osteoporosis

Latest studies show magnesium is more effective than calcium in preventing osteoporosis.

Progesterone Builds Bone

Estrogen stops bone from breaking down, but it is progesterone that actually builds it up.

Vitamin D And Osteoporosis

Women who live in the tropics have a lower incidence of osteoporosis, probably due to the Vitamin D produced in their bodies from the sunshine. This aids in the metabolism of calcium.

Overlooked Cause

An overactive thyroid can cause thinning of the bones.

Calcium Rip-Off

Latest studies show daily intake of extra calcium has no beneficial effect on the prevention of osteoporosis and hip fractures. It is more important to exercise daily to strengthen the muscles and connecting tissues of the bones. In addition it is necessary to take supplements of magnesium which allow for absorption of dietary calcium.

Too Much Of A Good Thing

When the skin is exposed to the sun, Vitamin D is manufactured in the body. Vitamin D is crucial for calcium absorption. If too much beta-carotene is in the system, it can block this process. Some people have trouble processing beta-carotene (this can be determined by a blood test).

Test For Bone Loss

Cross linking test (urine test) can determine the rate of bone loss.

Bank Your Bones

Most women don't consider taking supplemental calcium until they approach midlife. However, it is essential for women from age 15 to 35 to be sure to get enough calcium, magnesium and Vitamin D from food and supplements since bone production is highest during this time.

Bad Combination

Don't eat calcium-rich foods with whole grains since grains bind with calcium preventing its uptake. A cheese sandwich on whole wheat bread or cereal with milk might satisfy your appetite, but does not satisfy the body's calcium requirements.

UTERUS

Alleviate Fibroids

Uterine fibroids may be caused by an overabundance of estrogen that is not controlled by adequate progesterone. To relieve the condition use Progest cream.

Post-Menopausal Uterine Growths

Abnormal growths in the uterus after menopause are most likely due to factors other than fibroids and should be investigated.

PABA And Folic Acid Stimulate Fibroids

Women with fibroids should reduce their intake of PABA and folic acid because they are estrogen stimulators which affect the growth of these tumors.

Hysterectomy Lowers Endorphins

Hysterectomy can lead to depression due to lower production of endorphins (mood enhancers) post-operatively.

Ovaries Dependent On Uterus

The ovaries of women who have had simple hysterectomies (removal of uterus only) atrophy in two to three years because they lack specific hormones that were manufactured in the uterus.

Six Possible Aftereffects Of Hysterectomy

1. Urinary incontinence.
2. Decrease in sexual desire.
3. Imbalance between testosterone and estrogen.
4. Vaginal dryness.
5. Lower back pain due to severing of muscles, nerves and ligaments during surgery.
6. Increase in size of waist.

Overlooked Post-Hysterectomy Repair Procedure

When performing a hysterectomy, after the uterus and ovaries are removed, the surgeon should also incorporate a repair procedure so that the cervix or vagina does not prolapse in later years. In addition, muscles, ligaments and tendons should also be reattached at the same time. This is overlooked in many hysterectomies, causing the patient unnecessary long-term suffering.

Too Many Hysterectomies

A woman stands a 50 percent chance of having a hysterectomy by the age of 65. Each year 2000 women die from hysterectomies and 240,000 suffer major complications. Despite the fact that they are performed on only half the population (women), hysterectomies remain the most frequently performed major surgery.

Myoma Coagulation

A procedure called myoma coagulation cauterizes and destroys the blood supply to ovarian and uterine fibroids causing them to shrink remarkably. By utilizing this procedure, surgery and the hospital can often be avoided.

Shrink Uterine Fibroids

Pancreatic enzymes can be used to shrink uterine fibroids. The dosage is three (by Twinlab), three times a day between meals.

Alternatives To A Hysterectomy For Ovarian And Uterine Fibroids

Treatments other than hysterectomy for ovarian and uterine fibroids are:

- Micro surgery
- Laser surgery
- Myomectomy (removing fibroids only)
- Hormonal therapy
- Myoma coagulation

Although all but the hormonal therapy are surgical procedures, none are as drastic as a hysterectomy and you spend much less time in the hospital.

Understanding Your Pap Smear

50 percent of class 1 Pap smears disappear without treatment.

Class 2 and 3 Pap smears are not cancerous and are easily treated with high doses of folic acid which has close to a 100 percent cure rate.

Folic Acid Stems Cancer

Pap smears classified as grade 3 decreased to grade 1 or 2 when the women were treated with high amounts of folic acid (20 to 40 mg). In this strength, folic acid is available by prescription only. The folic acid available in the health food stores is such a low concentration that it would be necessary to take the contents of an entire bottle daily.

Treatment May Not Be Needed For Cervical Dysplasia

In cases of cervical dysplasia, 50 percent of the symptoms disappear without any treatment.

Abnormal Pap Smear

If a Pap smear shows atypical cervical cells, the following protocol, which is 100 percent effective, should be used daily:

- 50,000 I.U. Vitamin A
- 50,000 I.U. beta-carotene
- 10 mg folic acid (physician prescription necessary)
- GLA (evening primrose oil)

Atypical cells are often indicative of a precancerous condition, and the orthodox treatment for this is often methotrexate. The use of this chemotherapeutic agent here is just another example of orthodox overkill, and harmful, besides, because methotrexate blocks folic acid which is needed to alleviate the condition. Note: Other female cancers such as ovarian, uterine and breast *do* require the suppression of folic acid.

The Right Combination

Young women who have had hysterectomies are prescribed estrogen without progesterone. The orthodox reasoning is that, without the uterus, progesterone's protective factor is not needed. This is not true. When used alone, estrogen causes fluid retention. This can be alleviated by the addition of progesterone.

Rejected

Without adequate progesterone, the lining of the uterus will reject a fertilized egg or an implanted one.

Fiber Uptake

Increase fiber uptake to absorb excess estrogen if growing uterine fibroids are present.

Dairy Feeds The Tumor

Women with uterine fibroids should refrain from using dairy products, including butter, milk and cheeses (including cottage cheese and cream cheese, sour cream and yogurt). They should also avoid products which include dairy in their ingredients, such as baked goods, gravies and mashed potatoes. Dairy products are loaded with animal estrogens which enhance the growth of fibroids.

Overdoing

In hysterectomies, where only the uterus was diseased, 46 percent of healthy ovaries were also removed for no apparent reason.

Uterine Spasms

Women who suffered repeated miscarriages were found to be deficient in magnesium. This deficiency makes the uterus more susceptible to spasms.

Reproductive Organ Cancers

Soy Stymies Cancer

Soy products and beans contain genestein, a chemical that naturally deactivates the type of estrogen that can cause cancer in female organs.

Ovarian Cancer

Women who have had tubal ligations for the purpose of sterilization have one-third the risk of contracting ovarian cancer.

Vitamin E Soothes Inflamed Vagina

Women who have had radiation to the cervix or vagina may suffer from painful intercourse due to inflammation. This inflammation can be soothed by inserting three to four vitamin E capsules high into the vagina about 12 hours prior to sexual relations. The body acid will dissolve the capsules and the Vitamin E will repair the irradiated tissue.

SEXUALITY

Why He Wants To Buy You A Drink

Alcohol raises female testosterone levels which increases their sex drive.

A Downside Of Sex

Sexual activity is the most frequent cause of bladder infections in women.

Dry Vagina

Vitamin E suppositories are effective in lubricating a dry vagina.

Vaginal Infections

Women who have repeated vaginal infections of undetermined origin may be allergic to their partner's sperm. They should build up their immune systems by taking high doses of antioxidants, eating chemical-free organic foods, drinking distilled water, getting proper exercise and lowering their stress levels.

FEMALE YEAST PROBLEMS

Endometriosis

Candida (yeast infection) could be an underlying cause of endometriosis.

Yeast Causes Vaginitis

The underlying cause of vaginitis is infiltration of yeast (Candida) from the colon. Candida is exacerbated by antibiotics, birth control pills and Prednisone. If localized treatment of the vagina fails, systemic therapy is called for.

A Necessary Partner

Antibiotics are made from yeast. Women predisposed to Candida should be sure to take acidophilus when they have to take antibiotics. Acidophilus can be purchased in health food stores and is found in live cultures yogurt.

Help For Vaginal Yeast Infections

Boric acid suppositories are useful in treating vaginal yeast infections.

Supplements For Female Disorders

Flaxseed oil alleviates PMS, irregular periods and hot flashes.

Dandelion root is an effective diuretic for relieving water retention during menses.

Vitamin E suppositories relieve vaginal dryness.

An effective treatment for excessive menstrual bleeding is high dosages of Vitamin A in the form of fish liver oil, under the supervision of a nutritional doctor.

Tampon/Vaginitis Connection

Vaginal infections are often caused by tampons made of synthetic material. These tampons contain dioxen which is formulated by the bleaching process. Women should use only 100 percent cotton tampons which are bleached with peroxide. This type tampon may be difficult to obtain in the United States, but is readily available in Canada and England.

Soothing Bath

Improper douching may aggravate vaginitis. Instead, add three to four cups of cider vinegar to the bath water and soak for at least 20 minutes with legs apart so the water can flow into the inflamed area.

Forego Sexy Underwear

Fabrics that do not breathe, such as nylon, trap moisture and make an ideal breeding ground for yeast and parasites. Even nylon panties with a cotton panel hold too much moisture. Air circulation is important. Wear plain loose white cotton panties. Lingerie companies are beginning to make more attractive cotton panties.

20 Gallbladder

Prevention Of Gallstones

For the prevention of gallstones, have plenty of fiber in your diet, along with essential fatty acids and iodine, to keep cholesterol soluble (flowing in solution).

Gallbladder Pain

Fat consumption makes the gallbladder contract. This causes intense pain but *not* gallstones. Insoluble cholesterol (cholesterol that stagnates and does not flow) causes those.

Foods That Trigger Gallstones

Foods that can trigger gallstones and lead to a gallbladder attack are poultry, pork, beans and eggs (fatty foods). They cause the gallbladder to go into spasm. Bile is needed for fat metabolism and, if a stone blocks the duct, the bile will back up, causing severe pain.

Rapid Weight Loss

Too rapid a reduction in weight from dieting can lead to gallbladder problems since fat burnoff is activated through the liver.

Stonewalled

Gallstones are caused by the thickening of bile which flows through the gallbladder. The amino acid, L-Taurine, 1000 mg three times a day, can be used to help decrease the thickness of the bile which will become free-flowing, thereby lessening the possibility of stone production.

Vitamin C Deficiency

Be sure you are getting enough Vitamin C, at least 2000 mg daily. Vitamin C helps convert cholesterol into bile acids.

Risk Factors For Gallstones—The 4 F's

- Female
- Fat
- Fertile
- Forty

Four out of five people who get gallstones are women.

21 Gout

Low Purine Products

Patients with gout who have to eliminate purine-type foods (animal protein) from their diet can ingest dairy products which are low in purine. Fish oil, which is used as a treatment for gout, does not contain any protein.

High And Low Purine Products

Anyone suffering from gout should be aware that eggs and dairy are low in purine and beans and asparagus are high in purine.

Anti-Gout Diet

Do not consume any of the following:

- Alcohol
- Anchovies
- Asparagus
- Beans
- Fried foods
- Gravies
- Mushrooms
- Pastries
- Rich Desserts
- Sardines
- Shrimp
- Spices

22 Heart Disease

RISK FACTORS

Major Risk Factors

Most people who suffer fatal heart attacks in their 50's or 60's do not have any of the major risk factors (high cholesterol, high blood pressure, diabetes, obesity, high triglycerides, smoking and a sedentary lifestyle). The number one predictor of fatal heart attacks in this age group is job dissatisfaction. Number two is a low rating on a list of self-happiness factors. More deaths from heart attacks occur at 9 a.m. Monday mornings than on any other day of the week.

Iron Levels

High iron levels are a risk factor for heart disease.

Absence Of Risk Factors

Half of all heart attack victims do not have any risk factors at all.

Swollen Ankles

Swollen ankles, along with lower abdominal swelling, may be an indicator of a future heart condition.

Low Selenium Levels

Even though the Chinese and Finnish people consume a low fat diet and eat very minimal amounts of meat, they have a high degree of cardiovascular disease and heart attacks. This was due to extremely low levels of selenium in the diet. Overuse of chemical fertilizers has depleted their soil of selenium.

Most Heart Attacks Occur In The AM

More heart attacks occur in the morning hours from 5 to 10 AM because that is the time blood is thickest. Secretions of adrenalin and cortisol are also highest at this time of day. Wine consumed with the evening meal helps to thin the blood. This could be the reason for the French Paradox (why the French have a lower incidence of heart disease despite a diet loaded with rich food).

The Crack In The Wall

Diabetics suffer five times the incidence of cardiovascular disease because the high amounts of insulin in their bloodstream cause deterioration of the arteries, eventually leading to blockages. Insulin, a powerful hormone, causes microscopic tears in the internal arterial walls which then bleed. Cholesterol, triglycerides, platelets, protein and fibrinogens in the bloodstream are attracted to the torn areas of the arterial wall to seal it off. These materials then accumulate and eventually cause the occlusion.

Indicators Of Possible Heart Disease

- A diagonal crease in ear lobes.
- Baldness in the back of the head.
- Left-handed people have a higher risk of arrythmias and cardiac death.

Height Connection

Short men have a higher cardiac risk factor. This may stem from psychological insecurity.

Heart Disease Signal

Low blood pressure accompanied by heart pain is an indicator of heart disease.

Infant Size Predicts Coronary Health

Smaller-sized infants have a higher predisposition to heart disease later in life. Males who weighed 18 pounds or less at age one were fully three times more likely to have coronary heart disease later in life than those who weighed 26 pounds or more at that age. Therefore, it is possible that coronary heart disease is programmed during the early years.

Heart Failure

Heart failure is an indication that the heart muscle is weakening. Symptoms are:

- Shortness of breath.
- Swollen ankles.
- Awakening in the middle of the night and being unable to catch the breath.
- Fatigue.

Other Culprits

Cholesterol is not the only culprit causing heart disease. The others are high blood pressure, diabetes, smoking, lack of exercise, high triglycerides, high iron and genetics.

The Iron Culprit

Heart disease in women is not prevented by the hormone, estrogen. The protective factor is menstruation, which aids in the excretion of excess iron. Women who have had hysterectomies and were left with intact ovaries did not show any decrease in heart disease even though they were producing estrogen.

Hemachromatosis is a condition where too much iron is stored in the body. It is this stored iron which causes the problem by producing free radicals leading to the disruption of cell metabolism. A simple ferretin test can determine this level. High ferretin levels can be brought down by iron chelation or by donating blood.

Cholesterol And Heart Disease

Octogenerians Need Not Fear Cholesterol

At age 80 there is a higher incidence of heart disease in people with low cholesterol than with high cholesterol.

Cholesterol-Lowering Medications

Cholesterol is a marker of heart disease, not a cause.

All studies show cholesterol-lowering drugs do not prevent heart attacks. In fact, the death rate of patients who take the medication, compared to those who do not, is twice as high.

Insulin Imbalance

Insulin imbalance causes more heart attacks than high cholesterol levels.

Vitamin E Levels Crucial

Instead of testing for cholesterol levels, Vitamin E levels should be determined. Latest studies show that a deficiency in E levels has more of an impact on the risk of a heart attack than cholesterol levels do.

HDL

Heart disease is very rare in individuals with HDL readings higher than 65. Those whose HDL is below 35 are at risk, even if their total cholesterol is low.

Angiograms

Deadly Angiograms

To date, over 100,000 deaths have occurred from angiograms. More people have died from angiograms than died in the Vietnam War.

Angiograms Can Be Dangerous To Your Health

A thallium stress test is all that is needed to determine if the heart is receiving enough blood and oxygen. An angiogram is usually ordered instead and, in a high percentage of cases, it is merely a precursor to bypass surgery. During an angiogram, plaque can be dislodged and can cause an embolism in other vessels of the body, damaging vital organs.

Angiogram Interpretations

Show the results of your angiogram to 5 different cardiologists and chances are you will get 5 different opinions.

Angiogram interpretations are not even close to autopsy results.

Perfusion Study

A more important diagnostic tool than an angiogram is a perfusion study. This is a non-invasive procedure which, in addition to showing the coronary artery blood supply, also shows the amount of blood going to the entire heart muscle.

Digital Subtraction Test

A digital subtraction test for coronary evaluation gives the same results as a cardiac catheterization (angiogram). Both utilize dye, but the digital subtraction test is *not* an invasive procedure.

New Non-Invasive Procedure

MRA (Magnetic Resonance Angiography) is a new diagnostic procedure to determine the amount of plaque in coronary arteries. It is non-invasive (no dye has to be injected), unlike cardiac catheterization which can have dire side effects.

Heart Perfusion Test Overlooked

If the doctor insists on performing an angiogram on patients with chest pain, a perfusion test should be done. This test shows if enough blood is being pumped through the heart and into the system to handle the body's needs. If the perfusion test is normal and the cardiologist still insists bypass surgery is necessary, seek another opinion. In most cases where an angiogram shows blocked arteries and the patient has no symptoms, the body has developed collateral arteries which act as a natural bypass.

Collateral Circulation

Angiograms are often misleading because collateral circulation is not taken into consideration. Collateral circulation is the outgrowth of additional arteries that naturally bypass the occluded artery, bringing additional blood supply to the heart muscle. Collateral circulation can be so good that even if a coronary artery is blocked, the bypass is not needed.

ANGIOPLASTIES

Failure Of Angioplasties

One third of angioplasties fail in six months. After an angioplasty, the arterial wall is weakened and becomes susceptible to arteriosclerosis because the intima (the inner wall of the artery) is injured by scarring. This scar tissue develops rapidly and can reblock the artery.

Angina Returns

The recurrence rate of angina in patients who have undergone angioplasty is 50 percent in the first six months following the procedure. It is interesting to note that this procedure is performed by cardiologists, not surgeons.

Stop Arterial Blockage In Its Tracks

To stop the recurrence of arterial blockage following angioplasty, use fish oil (EPA-Omega 3) and borage oil (GLA-Omega 6).

BYPASS SURGERY

Statistics

- One out of 17 people die from bypass surgery, while only 1 in 75 die from the disease itself.
- The chance of a heart attack from bypass surgery is 5.5 percent.
- The chance of a heart attack from angioplasty (balloon procedure) is 2.5 percent.
- The chance of a heart attack from medication and a cardiovascular exercise program is 1 percent.

High-Tech Procedures Overrated

In 1993, 550,000 bypass procedures and 435,000 balloon angioplasties were performed at a total cost of $43 billion. There is very little evidence that these patients have a greater life expectancy than those on drug therapy.

Profitable Surgery

A New York study determined that only two percent of all bypass surgeries were necessary. The average bypass procedure generates $40,000.00 for the hospital alone.

Sham Surgery

This surgery was performed as part of a study by surgeons who believed the effectiveness of bypass surgery was overrated. The study showed that 56 percent of patients undergoing this sham heart operation (an incision similar to that used in bypass surgery is made on the chest) had relief of symptoms. And patients with this sham surgery were able to reduce their use of nitroglycerine.

Positive Side Effect Of Bypass

One reason that symptoms of angina improve following bypass surgery is that, during the operation, the surgeon severs the pericardium (sac covering the heart). This interrupts the nerve supply to the heart muscle so the patient does not feel the pain.

Ineffective Procedure

Bypass surgery does not prevent heart attacks. One in 17 patients dies from the surgery. One in 75 dies from the disease (CAST study performed by NIH). Death rates were lower in patients using conservative therapy (medication) than in those undergoing surgery.

Most of the one million angiograms performed yearly are inaccurate. Angiograms show a 2 dimensional view of blood circulating through the heart. Since the heart is a 3 dimensional structure, a 2 dimensional study shows only 66.6 percent of the true picture.

Angioplasties and bypasses cost millions of dollars per day for tests and treatments that are both inaccurate and ineffective most of the time. In fact, angiogram results are not even close to what the autopsies show.

Higher Bypass Failure Rate For Women

Due to women's smaller arteries and hearts, bypass surgery is not as successful for them as it is for men.

Asymptomatic Patients Should Nix Bypass Surgery

Asymptomatic patients (those with no symptoms of any heart disorder) who are diagnosed with clogged coronary arteries during a routine physical have a higher chance of survival by not undergoing bypass surgery. This surgery is effective in only five percent of asymptomatic patients and there is a six percent chance of dying during or immediately following the procedure. Also, the heart/lung machine used during the operation causes cognitive impairment (memory loss) in 50 percent of the cases. As the blood travels through the machine's metal tubing, it absorbs metal ions which get transported to the brain where they accumulate and cause destruction of essential brain cells.

More On The Heart/Lung Machine

When a patient is placed on the heart/lung machine during bypass surgery, it is almost the same as having a mini-stroke. Due to oxygen deprivation, brain cell capacity is diminished. This is why some people suffer memory loss and attention deficit syndrome following bypass surgery.

Bypass Surgery—Long-Term Outlook Dismal

Bypass surgery is one of the most unproven procedures in medicine. Latest studies have shown that long-term results in cardiac patients were the same whether or not this surgery was performed.

Overdone Procedures

Only two out of a hundred people with severe coronary artery blockage are at risk of having a heart attack.

Two controlled trials of bypass surgery performed in 1977 (CASS—Coronary Artery Surgery Study) and 1983 (Veterans Hospital Study) showed that this surgery does not prevent heart attack or death.

Blockages are reversible without bypass surgery.

Latest studies show that one third of angiograms are unnecessary.

Over-Intervention Fails

Studies done on patients with heart conditions at McGill University in Canada and at Stanford University in California show the following results:

	U.S.A.	Canada
Angiograms performed	55%	34%
Angioplasty	30%	13%
Bypass surgery	10%	4%
Recurrent rate of heart attacks	1%	1%
Deaths	12%	11%

Conclusion—More intervention does not necessarily produce better results.

HEART VALVES

Mitral Valve Prolapse

A diagnosis of mitral valve prolapse is no cause for alarm. The condition is a variation in one of the heart valves which billows slightly when the heart contracts. The heart is not abnormal in 99 percent of these patients. The valve does not deteriorate with time, does not interfere with the pumping of the heart and the person's longevity is not affected. Note: Statistics show mitral valve prolapse is less dangerous for a woman than for a man.

Antibiotics Overprescribed

Patients with mitral valve prolapse are advised to take antibiotics when dental work is being performed in order to prevent endocarditis (an inflammation of the lining of the heart). The use of antibiotics prophylactically is not always necessary, and there is always the possibility of a dangerous reaction to them. Use them for prevention of endocarditis only if the valve is thickened, or leaking, or if a murmur or regurgitation is present.

Replacement Heart Valves

Defective heart valves can be replaced with mechanical devices or with an animal's (usually a pig's) heart valves. In cases where a mechanical valve is utilized, patients must take blood thinners for the rest of their lives to prevent blood clots from forming on the valve. When an animal tissue valve is used, the problem does not occur.

Since the patient is on blood thinners with a mechanical valve, there is always a risk of bleeding. The advantage is that, in most cases, they do last longer than animal tissue valves.

PROMOTE CORONARY HEALTH

Fish And Olive Oil

In countries such as Greece, Italy and other Mediterranean areas where they consume large amounts of fish and olive oil, there is little heart disease.

Vegetarian Diet

A vegetarian diet can reduce angina pain by 91 percent.

Exercise

Daily exercise will reduce the risk of a heart attack by 60 percent.

Exercise Enhances Circulation

Exercise increases the number of blood vessels in the muscles, thereby increasing circulation, especially in the heart muscle.

Free Radical Scavenger

Vitamin E can reverse diet-induced arteriosclerosis. Vitamin E is a free radical scavenger which prevents the arterial walls from thickening. Free radicals in the molecules of the cells that line the arteries cause destruction, leading to abnormal cell growth in the interior walls of the arteries. As the arteries thicken, narrowing occurs, and they pick up debris from the blood supply, composed of cholesterol, triglycerides, fibrinogens, platelets and proteins.

Salmon Is Your Heart's Best Friend

Eating one-half pound of salmon four times a week will aid in eliminating the plaque which occludes the coronary arteries. Salmon contains eicosapentaenoic acid, also known as Omega 3, which helps produce anti-inflammatory prostaglandins.

Natural Chelator

Cayenne is a natural chelator. A combination of cayenne and garlic oil softens deposits in the arteries and flushes them out.

Although cayenne may cause a burning sensation in the digestive tracts of some individuals, it does not damage tissue.

Vitamin E Reduces Heart Disease

In a yearlong study, as few as 100 I.U.'s of Vitamin E daily reduced heart disease by 40 percent in women and 26 percent in men.

Beta-Carotene In Body Fat

High concentrations of beta-carotene in the body's adipose (fat) tissue reduces the risk of heart attacks.

Mediterranean Diet

The Mediterranean diet, found to increase longevity by lowering the death rate from heart conditions, consists of:

- 41 percent carbohydrates.
- 9 percent protein.
- 16 to 23 percent unsaturated lipids - extra virgin olive oil.
- 13 to 16 percent alcohol.

Liquid Form Of 2 Supplements Better

The liquid form of L-Carnitine and Co Q-10 are more effective than tablets or capsules of these for treating heart disease.

Open Up Your Arteries

To ease angina pain, take one Circu Cap by San Helois and two tablespoons of liquid alfalfa daily. This also eliminates symptoms of cold hands and feet.

Cardiac Arrhythmia

Cardiac arrhythmia can be controlled by using fish oil and flaxseed oil.

More Effective Aspirin Administration

Chewing an aspirin at the first sign of a heart attack is the quickest way of getting it into your system. Its blood-thinning effect could lessen the severity of the attack.

Regulate Heartbeat

Use selenium to help regulate heartbeat.

Heart Fluttering

To eliminate heart fluttering (PVC—premature ventricular contractions), induce vomiting or submerge the entire head in a basin of cold water.

ADDITIONAL HEART INFORMATION

Bundle Branch Block

Left bundle branch block (electrical activity that controls the heart) means there is an abnormality in the heart from scarring due to a previous heart attack. Right bundle branch block is usually benign.

Is It Angina Or A Heart Attack?

Most people do not know the difference between angina and a heart attack. Angina is usually relieved in a few minutes by resting. But when a heart attack occurs, the pain persists and increases, even at rest.

Simple Heart Test

Pain in the chest area that does not increase when walking is usually due to a digestive problem rather than a heart problem.

Nitroglycerine

Nitroglycerine used to alleviate angina pain causes dilation of blood vessels in the head, leading to headaches.

Rapid Heartbeat

Anemia can cause rapid heartbeat.

Heart Blockages

Most heart blockages are caused by only 30 to 40 percent occlusion.

Stress Test Too Stressful To Be Accurate

Treadmill tests to diagnose heart problems are inaccurate and overreactive due to the person's fear of the outcome of the test. If the same test was self-performed at home, the results would be entirely different.

Treatment Costs Disregarded

If a patient can be brought to a cardiac unit within four hours of a heart attack, medication can be administered to increase arterial blood flow to the heart. The State Of The Art drug used for this procedure in the United States is TPA (tissue plasminogen activator). In Canada, streptokinase is used. Streptokinase is one-sixth the cost of TPA.

Plaque Formation

The reason plaque forms in arteries and not in veins is that the blood pressure is higher in the arteries, causing them to crack and break down in unhealthy people.

Dilated Aorta

An enlarged or dilated aorta is not a dangerous condition.

Occluded Carotid Arteries

Occluded carotid arteries (the major arteries in the neck) can cause people to feel their heartbeat in their ears.

Arrhythmias

The first thing to look for in heart arrhythmias is a thyroid problem.

Beta Blockers

Beta blocker medications counteract the positive effects of exercise.

Heart Medications Backfire

In 1979 there were 322,000 hospital admissions for heart disease. In 1993 there were 877,000 admissions, almost a threefold increase. This increase is due to the over-prescribing and unnecessary administration of heart medication (beta blockers) such as Lopressor, Inderol, Tenormin, Corgard and Normadine.

Electric-Shock-Induced Rhythm Corrections

The success rate of electric-shock-induced rhythm corrections, used for treatment of heart palpitations, tachycardia, fibrillation and premature ventricular contractions, is only 20 percent.

Coronary Vessels

Whether 1, 2, or 3 vessels are blocked, the death rate is the same.

Arterial blockage does not necessarily determine the amount of blood flow. It is possible to have 100 percent blood flow through a 95 percent blocked artery and 20 percent flow through one with a 40 percent blockage.

There are 30,000 miles of blood vessels in the body and bypass surgery is performed on only 6 inches of these vessels.

Five times more blood flows through the arteries than is needed.

23 Hypertension (High Blood Pressure)

Lowering Blood Pressure May Be Dangerous To Your Health

In certain cases, people over age 70 with diastolic blood pressure (the lower reading) of 90 to 95, should not receive treatment because their systems have adapted to this level. Lowering their pressure to 75 or 80, could impede their energy levels and also cause problems such as weakness, fatigue, and dizziness that could lead to falls.

Blood Pressure Medication Bends Penis

Medication to lower blood pressure can cause Perrones Disease, a fibrosis or thickening of the outer capsule of the penis, causing the organ to bend at an uncomfortable angle. This can lead to uncomfortable intercourse.

Safe Licorice

The herb, licorice, retains sodium in the body which can cause fluid retention and lead to high blood pressure. Be sure to use only deglycyrrhizinated licorice.

Decreasing Salt Intake Overrated

Studies have shown that using less salt in the diet reduces blood pressure only four percent.

Slightly Higher Blood Pressure In Elderly No Cause For Alarm

A slight elevation of blood pressure in individuals over 60 is no cause for alarm. As one ages, the arteries lose flexibility and they narrow, allowing less blood to enter the heart muscle. A slight elevation in pressure, to allow the heart to pump enough blood to adequately nourish all parts of the body, is nature's way of compensating for this inadequacy. Therefore, slightly higher blood pressure in older people should not be lowered by medication, but by natural methods, such as dieting if overweight and incorporating meditation and biofeedback into their daily routine. Use supplements such as Vitamin C and B^6, L-Taurine and the herbs garlic and Hawthorne berries.

Ginseng

Ginseng normalizes blood pressure, increasing it when it's too low and decreasing it when too high.

Low Blood Pressure

Licorice root and sodium (simple salt) will raise low blood pressure.

Medication Backfires

Twenty-five to 40 percent of those told they have high blood pressure actually do not, and they are mistakenly given unnecessary medication which causes other problems, specifically loss of sodium and potassium through the overprescribing of diuretics. Sodium and potassium are essential minerals needed by your body for controlling the electrical activity of the heart and central nervous system, and the loss of these minerals can cause disturbances in heart rhythm. Diuretics also deplete magnesium, causing spasms of coronary arteries and leading to occlusions and possible heart attacks.

Sugar Worse Than Salt

One cause of high blood pressure is sugar, not salt, consumption. Sugar causes the production of insulin which causes the body to retain its own manufactured sodium. It is *this* sodium, not dietary salt, that is the cause of high blood pressure.

Stay Out Of The Cold

The lower the temperature, the higher the blood pressure. More blood clots are produced in cold weather because fibrinogen, which is responsible for blood clotting, rises in cold weather.

Effect Of Positional Changes

Ortho Static Hypotension is a decrease in blood pressure that occurs with a change in position. It can occur when doing something as simple as leaning over to tie one's shoes. This can be detrimental for anyone with low blood pressure because it could make them feel lightheaded or dizzy.

Chrysanthemum Tea

Chrysanthemum tea lowers blood pressure.

Blood Pressure Medication

Certain blood pressure medications can raise cholesterol.

Don't Block Your Channel

Calcium channel blockers given for hypertension, such as Cardizem, Isoptin and Procardia, may raise the risk of a heart attack. According to a recent study at the University of Washington, patients with high blood pressure increased their risk of having a heart attack 60 percent if they were on calcium channel blockers.

This medication slows down the contraction of the heart muscle to protect it from overexertion. If a person taking channel blockers performs an activity such as vacuuming, or gets overexcited at a movie, overexertion of the heart muscle could occur. The heart still has to strain against the contractual lowering effect of the medication and this can actually cause the blood pressure to rise so much that a heart attack would be imminent.

Blood/Brain Barrier Fails

Prevailing cytotoxins (substances that inhibit proper cell functioning) in the blood are prevented from entering the brain by a natural barrier (blood/brain barrier). This protective barrier will fail if a stroke occurs because of high blood pressure. In the body's effort to increase blood flow to the brain, the barrier fails, allowing cytotoxins to enter the brain, causing inflammation and infection.

Magnesium Levels Crucial

One of the main causes of hypertension is a dilated artery going into spasm and constricting which limits the amount of blood to the heart. Magnesium relaxes the spasmodic muscle surrounding the arteries.

Although blood levels of magnesium can be high in the serum, that does not indicate adequate amounts are in the cells. High levels in the serum indicate magnesium is spilling from the cells and lowering the amount needed by them. Note: Blood levels of magnesium in the cell should be investigated.

Downside Of Licorice Root

Licorice root increases blood pressure by lowering potassium levels. When potassium levels are low, sodium levels rise, causing fluid retention which leads to a rise in blood pressure. Use only the deglycyrrhizinated form of licorice.

Beware Of Lasix

The effects of Lasix, a drug used for controlling blood pressure, last only six hours. Lasix depletes Vitamin B^1 which can cause beriberi and/or circulatory problems leading to heart malfunction. Low B^1 levels lead to higher sodium levels and fluid retention. Vitamin B^1 aids in improving the blood ejection factor in the heart by 22 percent.

Medication Is A Headache

Beta blockers, which lower blood pressure, can cause headaches in older patients because blood circulation to the brain is diminished.

Coronary Predictor

Blood pressure readings should be taken in the ankle as well as the arm. If the readings are far apart, it may be a predictor of future heart condition from blockage.

Protect Against Strokes

Vitamin C levels are a higher determinant for strokes than high diastolic blood pressure.

24 Kidney And Bladder

Improving Kidney Function

Chelation therapy is extremely effective for improving kidney function.

Kidney Problem Indicator

High magnesium readings in the blood may be indicative of kidney problems.

Ibuprofen

Extended use of ibuprofen can cause kidney failure.

Cayenne Red Pepper

Cayenne red pepper will help eliminate the burning, bleeding and frequency associated with urinary problems.

Fluids Essential

A high BUN reading may be due to not having consumed enough fluids. Patients could be treated with dangerous medication when simply drinking more water is all that is necessary.

Revelations Of Excised Tumors

Thirty to 50 percent of kidney tumors recur after removal. Perhaps it would be wise to study the 50 to 70 percent of patients whose tumors do not recur and see what is different about them.

Interstitial Cystitis

Interstitial cystitis is a condition where the nerves that are used in emptying the bladder do not work (neurogenic bladder). Infection often occurs and it is often caused by allergies or yeast infections. An overgrowth of yeast will irritate and inflame the bladder.

Treatment For Bladder Infections

Vitamin C is the best treatment for bladder infections. It works by changing the pH of the urine to a higher acid level.

Protect The Bladder

Cranberry and goldenseal bind up the receptor cells in the bladder, protecting it from the bacteria that can cause cystitis.

Cranberry Extract

Use cranberry extract instead of the juice for bladder infections because the amount of cranberry juice necessary to be effective is one quart daily, and it has a high content of sugar.

Another Cause Of Bladder Infection

The diaphragm, used for contraception, can lead to bladder infections.

Stop The Leak

Artemesia Annui (a health food store item) can help control urinary incontinence.

Don't Get Dilated

Many women with cystitis have their urethras dilated in order to facilitate emptying the bladder. This can damage the muscle needed for urinary control and lead to incontinence.

Back/Bladder Connection

Bladder problems in women are often due to lumbar instability (low back problems such as pinched nerve, herniated disc and muscle spasms) which can cause nerve and blood flow interruption. The following exercises exacerbate lumbar instability and should be avoided.

- High impact aerobics
- Jogging
- Nordic Track
- Running
- Stairmaster
- Weightlifting

More On Interstitial Cystitis

Interstitial cystitis, a severe bladder infection with no known cure, can be alleviated by taking high amounts of Vitamin A—100,000 I.U.'s daily but, due to the possible of liver toxicity, this must be under a doctor's supervision. Also, the addition of 35 percent food grade hydrogen peroxide (not the 3 1/2 percent solution) will facilitate the uptake of oxygen into the bladder cells. 35 percent food grade hydrogen peroxide should be taken in the following manner.

Week 1 —Add 1/4 teaspoon to 1 quart of distilled water.
Week 2 —Add 1/2 teaspoon to 1 quart distilled water.
Week 3 —Add 3/4 teaspoon to 1 quart distilled water.
Week 4 —Add 1 teaspoon to 1 quart distilled water.
Drink 1 eight ounce glass every 4 hours.

Bladder Hyperplasias

High doses of Vitamin A have been successful in reversing hyperplasias in the bladder. Since these high doses can be toxic, patients should be monitored by blood tests.

25 Lupus

Vitamin E Stymies Lupus

It has been shown that high amounts of Vitamin E (2000 to 3000 I.U.'s daily) are beneficial for controlling lupus.

Molybdenum And Lupus

Molybdenum, a mineral, aids in repairing the defect in an enzyme that causes lupus.

Food Allergies And Lupus

Lupus sufferers should be examined for food allergies.

Male Hormones Benefit Female Lupus Sufferers

Women with lupus have extremely low levels of testosterone and androgens. Raising these levels stimulates the immune system. Testosterone and DHEA help protect men against some autoimmune diseases such as lupus. Therefore treatment with testosterone and DHEA should be given to females who contract these diseases.

26 Migraines

Absorption Of Medication

Patients with migraine headaches may not absorb orally administered medication. If oral medication is not effective, use suppositories instead.

Progest Cream

Progest cream applied topically will relieve migraines in women.

Food Allergies And Migraines

Migraine headaches are often due to a food allergy. An elimination diet will identify what foods are causing the problem.

Foods To Avoid

Avoid high tyramine foods to prevent migraine headaches. The following foods are high in tyramines.

- Avocados
- Bananas
- Beer
- Canned figs
- Cheese
- Chicken livers
- Chocolate
- Cola
- Eggplant
- Fava Beans
- Liver
- Pickled herring
- Raisins
- Soy sauce
- Tea
- Wine
- Yeast extract
- Yogurt

Alleviate Migraines

Acupuncture, fish oil and feverfew (an herb) are useful to alleviate migraines.

Warm Hands

Warm your hands to treat migraines. It improves blood circulation.

Reduce Histamine Levels

Alka Seltzer Gold makes the blood more alkaline, helping to reduce the histamine levels that cause vasospasms leading to migraines.

Sweet Headache

Nutra-Sweet has been implicated as a cause of migraine headaches. It precipitates an allergic reaction which causes over-expansion and contraction of arteries in the skull, leading to headaches.

Salad Bar Migraines

Migraine sufferers should attempt to keep their systems alkaline by using raw vegetables and fruits organically grown. They should be especially wary of salad bars since sulfites are often used to maintain a fresh appearance.

Benefit Of Menopause

During the menstrual cycle, hormonal changes can precipitate migraine headaches. Many women who suffer from migraines find they decrease after menopause.

The Right Juice

Orange or grapefruit juice may precipitate a migraine headache. Carrot and celery juice help relieve migraine headaches.

Keep Eating

Wide swings in blood sugar may cause a migraine attack. In order to keep blood sugar levels stable, it is better to consume several small meals and eat between meals rather than eat three large meals.

27 Multiple Sclerosis

Diagnosing Multiple Sclerosis

If a patient still has symptoms of multiple sclerosis following a negative MRI, a spinal tap should be performed for a diagnosis.

Swank Diet

The SWANK diet (no animal fats) can alleviate symptoms of multiple sclerosis. The SWANK diet consists of foods containing essential fatty acids such as fish and vegetables and polyunsaturated oils such as safflower, sunflower and soybean.

Causes Of Multiple Sclerosis

Some possible causes are:

- Inhalation of platinum from catalytic convertors in automobiles.
- Electromagnetic fields.
- Mercury in silver fillings
- Material used in root canals.
- Hypoglycemia.

Orthodox Treatment

Orthodox treatment for multiple sclerosis does not cure the disease, merely slows it down.

Bee Venom

Bee venom therapy is effective for treating multiple sclerosis. The American Apitheraphy Society in Hartland Four Corners, VT, can tell you more about it. Their toll-free number is 1-800-823-3460.

28 Parkinson's Disease

Vitamin E

Oxidation of neurons (cell death) in critical brain cells can cause Parkinson's Disease. Vitamin E (an antioxidant) stops this.

L-Dopa And B^6

Parkinson's patients taking L-Dopa should not take therapeutic doses of Vitamin B^6 as this counteracts the effect of the medication.

Dangerous Flu Vaccine

Check to be sure mercury has not been used as a preservative in flu vaccine. It could cause Parkinson's disease.

Diet For Parkinson's Patients

Utilize a low protein, high carbohydrate diet for Parkinson's Disease since proteins interfere with nerve transmitters.

29 Prostate Problems And Male Conditions

Balding Patterns

Balding patterns can be indicative of physical problems.

- Top center of forehead—lung problems.
- Sides of forehead—kidney and bladder problems.
- Crown of head—heart and liver problems.
- Back of head—intestinal problems.

Underweight Men

A man's inability to gain weight may be due to low testosterone levels.

Indispensable Testosterone

Testosterone is a muscle enhancer which aids in the function of the heart muscle. It also helps the smooth muscles of the arteries to regulate blood pressure and prevent arteriosclerosis.

Leydig acid in the testicles produces testosterone. The prostate gland converts the testosterone to dehydrotestosterone (DHT), a much more potent form. This conversion in the prostate is activated by the enzyme, #5 alpha reductase. The drug, Proscar, reduces the amount of DHT produced.

Testosterone levels decline with age. Benign prostatic hypertrophy, a condition that develops as a man ages, is known as andropause, the male equivalent of menopause.

If an insufficient amount of testosterone is produced in the testicles, the muscle surrounding the prostate gland will not absorb enough of it. This will cause the prostate to become dysfunctional which will lead to fibrosis. This muscle surrounding the prostate plays an important role in helping the urethra dilate. (The urethra is the tube in the prostate and penis that urine flows through.) If this process fails, constriction occurs, causing an interrupted urine flow.

A testosterone deficiency will lead to a compensatory enlargement of the prostate gland. It is actually a deficiency, not a surplus, of testosterone that causes an enlargement of the prostate. Before any procedures are instituted or any medication is administered, blood levels of testosterone should be determined.

Treating men with Lupron, an antihormonal medication which slows the release of testosterone from the testicles, also prevents the testosterone from going to the heart muscle and leads to a weakened heart and eventual heart attack. Yet, this is still the treatment of choice for benign prostatic hypertrophy.

A better approach would be to raise testosterone levels in older men to offset this deficiency. Note: This applies only to BPH, not to cancer of the prostate.

Ulcer Medication Swells Male Breast

Some ulcer medications taken for longer than six months can cause breast enlargement in males.

ENLARGED PROSTATE

Soy Products

Soy products produce natural chemicals that block the effect of activated testosterone on enlarged prostate tissue.

Antihistamines

Antihistamines can lead to prostate enlargement. (See page 220 for supplements to alleviate enlarged prostate).

Disturbed Urine Flow

Older men with enlarged prostates tend to get cystitis due to incomplete emptying of their bladders. The enlarged prostate exerts pressure on the urethra, preventing the bladder from emptying completely.

Lupron's Side Effects

Lupron, a drug given for prostate problems, often causes night sweats.

Proscar Vs Saw Palmetto Berries

Fewer than 37 percent of patients on Proscar experienced clinical improvement in urinating in a six month period. Men taking Saw Palmetto berries (an herb) had a 90 percent improvement in four to six weeks.

- Proscar costs $75.00 per month.
- Saw Palmetto berries cost $24.00 per month, and can be purchased in a health food store.
- Proscar reduces libido.
- Saw Palmetto berries stimulate libido.

Prostate Medication Causes Birth Defects

Men who impregnate their partners while taking Proscar, a prostate shrinking medication, may have a child with birth defects.

Hair's The Way

External application of saw palmetto berries can alleviate hair loss by acting as a 5 Alpha Reductase (enzyme) inhibitor. This enzyme causes testosterone produced in the testicles to convert to the more active form (dehydrotestosterone) which causes the hair follicles to shrink. American Indians and Eskimos do not suffer from hair loss because they have much less 5 Alpha Reductase on their skin.

Stef Revitalizing Compound is a useful product containing saw palmetto berries in combination with other natural hair growth stimulants and is available in Canada. Contact Mike Stratis at Stef International in Toronto (1-800 327-4283).

Enhancing The Wrong Muscle

Arginine, often used to enhance muscle growth, produces high amounts of nitric acid in the system. Too much nitric acid can cause problems with erections.

Supplements To Alleviate Enlarged Prostate

- Zinc
- Manganese
- Vitamin E
- Pycnogenol
- Amino acids—glutamic acid, glycine and alanine

Medication Slows Urine

Antihistamines can have an adverse effect on the prostate slowing down urination.

Heat Treatment Shrinks Enlarged Prostate

Hyperthermia for enlarged prostate increases blood flow to the area, supplying the cells with nutrients and oxygen which allows the gland to revert to normal size.

Aftereffects Of Cryoblation

Cryoblation (a freezing procedure) for enlarged prostate has a 95 percent immediate success rate. Although this is an effective procedure, it does produce scar tissue which at a later date could make the original problem worse by causing urine retention.

PROSTATE CANCER

Radical Prostatectomy

The three side effects of a radical prostatectomy are leakage of urine, pain and infertility.

Cryosurgery Merely Palliates

Cryosurgery for prostate cancer or enlarged prostate works by freezing and destroying the cells. This shrinks the prostate's size. Men must be aware this treats only the symptoms and the cancer can return if the patient does not make changes in his lifestyle, diet, vitamin and mineral intake and exercise program.

Antihormonal Drug

Fludimide, an antihormonal drug used to treat prostate cancer, causes diarrhea.

Side Effects Of Prostate Surgery

Prostate surgery has severe side effects such as, back problems caused by the severing of sacral nerves, colon problems, erection problems and incontinence.

Hot Flashes

Lupron, used as an antihormonal drug to treat prostate cancer, has side effects of hot flashes and anemia.

Proscar Slows Libido

Proscar use in treatment of prostate cancer can cause minor impotence.

Better Left Alone

Autopsy results on men 60 to 70 years old showed prostate cancer in 46 percent of them. Yet the disease only affects one percent of the male population. Therefore, early detection is bad because it leads to early treatment of men who will not be affected by the disease and who must suffer pain and debilitation of unnecessary procedures.

Don't Concentrate The Pesticides

When juicing therapy is used to treat prostate cancer, be sure only organic fruits and vegetables are used. When you juice inorganic produce, the pesticides become concentrated.

Toxins In Cancer Cells

High amounts of pesticides, herbicides, DDT, mercury and heavy metals are found in the prostate cancer cells and not in adjoining normal cells.

PSA (Prostate Specific Antigen) Test For Prostate Cancer

Misleading Prostate Test

PSA, a blood test for prostate cancer, can also be elevated due to benign prostate enlargement or subsequent to a palpating rectal examination. The test should be performed prior to the palpation.

Ups And Downs Of PSA

TURP (transuretheral resection of the prostate), is a procedure where the center part of the prostate is removed to reduce the size of the gland. This reduction in the amount of prostate tissue will lower the PSA reading. PSA is produced by both normal and cancerous tissue, but a cancerous prostate makes more of it. A slight elevation in the level could be due to an enlarged prostate, not necessarily a cancerous one.

PSA Determinates

Men with enlarged prostates should have a PSA density test, since the results of the test take into consideration the volume of the gland. For example, if a man has a reading of 5 (4 is considered normal), and his prostate is larger than another man's with a 5 reading, chances are the first man's ratio is lower and he has less probability of cancer.

High PSA Reading

A PSA reading over 25 indicates prostate cancer has metastasized to other parts of the body.

Elevated PSA Does Not Always Indicate Cancer

An elevated PSA reading may not necessarily be caused by cancer. It could be due to a yeast infection, bacteria, inflammation, irritation or allergies. Patients with high PSA readings should be further evaluated by a holistic physician before serious surgical procedures requiring hospitalization are instituted.

False Positive PSA

A high PSA may also be caused by a urinary tract infection and/or parasites. These two conditions should be ruled out before ordering further testing or alarming the patient.

PENIS

Best Time To Perform A Circumcision

Vitamin K, a blood coagulator, is produced naturally in the body and is highest on the eighth day of life. Therefore that is the best time to perform a circumcision as there will be less bleeding.

Bloody Semen

Blood found in semen following ejaculation is usually no cause for alarm. It is generally from a benign condition called hematospermia.

Beneficial Side Effect Of Prozac

One side effect of Prozac is that it stops ejaculation. It is now being recommended as a treatment for premature ejaculation.

Yohimbe Aids Love Life

Yohimbe works on the central nervous system's receptor sites that control erection.

Bodybuilders

Bodybuilders who use arginine and ornithine, two substances which release growth hormones, may suffer side effects such as impotence, diabetes and breast enlargement (gynecomastia).

Impotence May Be Medically Induced

Drugs that can cause impotence are anti-hypertension medication, diuretics, alpha blockers, beta blockers, tranquilizers, anti-depressants and nasal decongestants.

Impotent Cyclists

Cyclists who are impotent may be irritating the perineal (testicular) area by constantly jolting it with a hard seat. The condition is reversible.

Impotence Ends Up In Your Head

Impotence starts out as a physical problem caused by poor circulation to the penile area. Then it becomes a psychological problem when the man loses his ability to perform sexually.

Impotence Predicts

Impotence in a male usually precedes death by 20 years. Impotence generally foreshadows a future heart condition.

Leave Well Enough Alone

Complications of the penis extension procedure are:

- Infection.
- Formation of scar tissue that may distort the extension.
- Loss of sensation.
- Encapsulation of the added fat leading to a lumpy organ.

Following the procedure, the man must abstain from sex for one month. Pain will be present for two to three weeks. The cost is in the $6,000.00 range.

Continuous Erection

Priapism is a continuous erection as a consequence of disease and is not related to sexual arousal. It could be caused by a blood clot and could lead to gangrene of the penis.

Bent Penis

Peyronie's disease (a painful condition where part of the sheath of fibrous connective tissue within the penis thickens, causing the organ to bend at an angle during erection) can be treated with high doses of PABA (12 grams spaced throughout the day). PABA in high doses acts as an anti-fibroic agent.

Peyronie's And Chelation

Chelation therapy is beneficial in removing calcification from the penis in cases of Peyronie's Disease.

FERTILITY

Don't Always Trust A Vasectomy

In a few cases, men who have had vasectomies still produced enough sperm to impregnate a female.

Sperm Quality

Sperm quality decreases in hot weather.

INFERTILITY

Check For Varicoceles

Infertile men should be checked for a varicocele (varicose vein in the testicle). A varicocele makes the testicles warm due to the presence of an abnormal amount of blood. Heat decreases sperm production, leading to infertility.

Undescended Testicles

An undescended testicle could be sterile when it finally descends.

Keeping Cool Helps Make Babies

Men attempting to become fathers, should avoid hot tubs.

And they should wear boxer shorts instead of jockey shorts to keep the testicles from getting too warm.

Sperm Stimulator

Use L-Carnitine for impotence and infertility. 3000 mg daily increases sperm count and motility after four months.

Endangered Procreation

The mean concentration of sperm has decreased in the last 20 years from 89 million per milliliter to 60 million per milliliter.

The quality of the sperm has also declined and their activity has lessened.

Author's note: This phenomenon is partially caused by the overproduction of synthetic chemicals which are destroying the quality of the air that people breathe. This is an example of the greed of a few determining the survival of our civilization.

Sperm Count Down

There has been a 50 percent reduction in sperm count and motility in the past 50 years. A recent study showed that workers exposed to petrochemicals were the most affected. *To increase sperm count,* use the following supplements daily:

- L-Carnitine, 3000 mg
- L-Arginine, 4000 mg
- Zinc, 50 mg

But I Had A Vasectomy!

One of every 2000 vasectomies fail.

Prostate Size

Normal prostate size should be approximately 23 cubic centimeters.

Hearing Loss

Men lose their hearing 30 years before women.

30 Psychological And Emotional

Anti-Depressant Drugs

All anti-depressant drugs become addictive and then the addiction becomes more of a problem than the original depression.

How To Eliminate A Panic Attack

Deep breathing will eliminate most panic attacks. Inhaling oxygen lessens the acidity of the body. Acid conditions inflame nerve cells, specifically in the brain, causing feelings of apprehension, anxiety or panic. This can be alleviated by changing the pH of the body to a more alkaline state. Calcium and magnesium added to the diet are natural ways to acquire higher alkalanity.

Mood Affects Immune System

Interleukin 2, and alpha interferon (immune system stimulants manufactured in the body) are increased when a person is happy and decreased when he or she is depressed or under stress.

Perception Of Life

Once your perception of life is altered through natural means (positive thinking, determination, conviction and the use of meditation), then biology will respond positively.

Love Yourself

Vanity can be good for your health. Those who take pride in how they look tend to have a stronger desire to take care of themselves.

Friends For Health

People with a sense of loneliness and isolation have three to five times the mortality rate of those with a sense of connection and family. People need bonding and social support systems for good health.

Test Before Prescribing

Doctors should test for neurotransmitter levels before prescribing antidepressant drugs.

Neurotransmitters are substances such as dopamine, seratonin, neuroepinephrine and adrenalin that transmit nerve impulses across a synapse. The most effective supplement to increase these levels is tryptophan, which was removed seven years ago by the FDA. It has not been allowed back, although other substances such as Perrier and Tylenol, which were found to be contaminated, have been allowed back.

Other supplements which can increase neurotransmitter levels are GABA plus by Twinlab, St. John's Wort (an herb), Tyrosene (an amino acid) Vitamins B^1, B^6 and B^{12} and a combination of Valerian root, hops, skullcap and passion flower.

Put On A Happy Face

When you act happy, you raise your levels of serotonin (a mood elevator). When you act sad, you lower the levels.

Hyperactive Children

Ritalin, a drug prescribed for hyperactive children, may cause addictive behavior later in life, including street drug addiction.

Hypnotize Your T Cells

The mind/body connection is so powerful that hypnotic suggestion can trigger a rise in T cells (immune system).

Don't Grieve Too Long

A normal mourning period lasts about six weeks. If severe grieving lasts much longer, the person should be treated for depression by an orthomolecular psychiatrist.

Laugh Your Way To Wellness

Laughter lowers stress hormones (cortisol and adrenalin) and raises endorphins (the body's natural chemicals for pain relief). It also lowers high blood pressure and the heart rate.

Sensory Digestion

Digestion refers to more than food. It also pertains to digestion of everything you see, hear, smell and touch.

Blame Yourself

People who do not adhere to recommended holistic principles blame the practitioner rather than themselves when they do not get results from the program.

Ions—The Ignored Treatment

A negative ionizer is effective in treating SAD (seasonal affective disorder), caused by a lack of sunlight in winter combined with low negative ions in the atmosphere. Bright light has been used as a treatment, but the impact of ionization had been ignored. For further information, read *The Ion Effect* by Soyka.

Chelation Therapy

Chelation therapy is effective in the treatment of senile dementia because it helps to clear out heavy metal plaque in the tiny capillaries of the brain.

Have You Lived Before?

Brian Weiss, M.D., a physician and author of *Many Lives Many Masters* and *Through Time Into Healing,* is having excellent results using past life regression to treat patients with illnesses and psychological problems. This process works by bringing traumatic experiences from a person's past life into awareness and then resolving the problems.

The patient is hypnotized and regressed to the time in a past life when the trauma occurred. People who have a difficult time making decisions may have made a wrong decision in a past life and fear repeating it. According to this theory, birthmarks are scars or trauma from a past life.

Schizophrenia

Schizophrenia has been shown to intensify in the spring, because of allergies attacking the brain. Most schizophrenics are allergic to milk or wheat.

Danger Of Diet Soda

Diet sodas contain a large amount of phenylalanine, an amino acid which has a tendency to overstimulate brain neurotransmitters. This overstimulation can cause panic attacks, hyperactivity and tremors. It imbalances the body's amino acids.

A Little Stress Will Do You Good

Short-term stress can actually jump start the immune system, but long-term stress will burn it out and lead to illness.

Tranquilizers

75 percent of all tranquilizers are prescribed for women.

Breathe In The Good

When under stress, breathing slows and makes the body more acid, which in turn exacerbates the stress. Deep diaphragmatic breathing exercises daily will alleviate this condition.

Reality And Illusion

The body reacts the same to a real or imaginary experience. (Example—nightmares.)

Heart Transplant Changes Personality

A person who receives a heart transplant takes on some of the personality of the donor.

Communicate With Your Immune System

Keeping a journal can enhance the immune system. One technique is to write a letter to the disease.

Healthy Thoughts

Anticipation of a pleasant event can enhance the immune system.

Don't Bury Anger

Sickness is caused by people burying their anger and dying inside.

Unproven Long-Term Drug Therapy

Most antidepressant drugs introduced in the late 50's were tested only for short-term use, but have been used for long-term therapy.

Feeling Depressed? It May Be Your Medication

Seventy-five percent of all drugs in the PDR (Physician's Desk Reference) list depression as a possible side effect.

Female Fat Blocks Love

Extremely obese women may have gained the weight as a defense against a relationship.

31 Shingles

Miracle Hot Stuff

Creams and ointments containing cayenne red pepper extract are useful for relieving the pain and burning associated with peripheral neuropathy or shingles. Peripheral neuropathy is caused by demyelinization of the nerve coating. You can make your own ointment by combining cayenne pepper with vinegar and enough water to make a paste. Along with this topical application, vitamins B^{1}, B^{12}, B^{6} and folic acid aid the healing process.

Onions

Rub a slice of onion on shingle sores to relieve the itching.

Shingles Aftermath

Post-herpetic neuralgia (following shingles) can be treated effectively with injections of B^{1}, B^{12} and AMP (adenosine mono phosphate)

Vitamin E Oil

Rub Vitamin E oil into shingle eruptions to reduce scarring.

32 Sinus And Colds

Sinus Flush

For basic sinus hygiene, dissolve 1/2 teaspoon of salt in 8 ounces of warm water. Inhale through the nose, allow the solution to drip into the throat and expectorate. This will keep the sinuses clean and prevent sinus flare-ups. Salt kills bacteria.

Ineffective And Dangerous Cold Medications

Antihistamines are not effective for treating colds. They are for relief of allergies. Decongestants dry up secretions, but don't cure the cold any faster. Side effects are overstimulation, increase in blood pressure, and urinary retention in men with prostate problems.

Stimulate Killer Cells

Lysine, 500 mg three times daily on an empty stomach, has antiviral capabilities. Colds are viral infections.

Garlic increases the activity of natural killer (NK) cells.

Grandma Was Right

Hot tea or chicken soup stimulates nasal secretions. If the speed of the secretions is stimulated and a virus lands on the mucous blanket, it will be transported away from the upper respiratory tract by swallowing and will be subsequently destroyed in the digestive tract. This action prevents the virus from penetrating the mucous layer and entering the cell where it can cause a common cold. Cold beverages decrease the speed of nasal mucous secretions. Chicken soup is the most effective hot beverage.

Sweat It Out

Fever and flu symptoms can be reduced by using the herb, boneset. It is a natural diaphoretic which induces sweating, opens the pores and allows the heat to dissipate, thereby preventing it from building up to too high a level.

Natural Antihistamines

Most sinus problems are due either to environmental or food allergies. Vitamin C and Quercetin (a bioflavanoid) are natural antihistamines.

Herbal Tea For Colds, Sinusitis And Postnasal Drip

Steep two Pau D'Arco tea bags and two Maté tea bags in one cup of hot water for 10 minutes. Drink one cup of this tea three times a day.

Overlooked Sinus Remedy

Sinus infections are often precipitated by an allergic reaction, causing an overproduction of histamine. The herb nettle can help lessen histamine production. Nettles produce a small amount of histamine which acts as a desensitizing agent.

Duck Your Cold

Oscillococcinum, a homeopathic remedy for colds and flu, effectively stimulates the immune system to destroy the invading viruses and bacteria. This preparation is derived from the ground-up internal parts of ducks.

33 Skeletal System

Facial Tics

Check the first cervical vertebra (atlas) and spine alignment for tics and spasms in the face.

Muscle Cramps

Quinine water relaxes muscle cramping.

Balance The Body

When there are problems in a leg stemming from neurological causes (cramping, pins and needles, numbness), the opposite arm must be investigated and treated in order to balance the system. Use of neural organization techniques (chiropractic, acupressure) is recommended. Adjusting the opposite arm corrects the imbalanced circuit to the brain and leg.

Knee Problems

Most knee problems are caused by the feet pronating (rolling out) or supinating (rolling in). Proper running shoes can prevent the problem.

Lysine Helps Rebuild Bone

Lysine, an amino acid not generally prescribed as a bone enhancer, aids in the absorption of calcium from the intestines, improving calcium's retention in the body, and making it an effective component in rebuilding bone tissue.

Danger Of Prednisone

Prednisone should not be given to people with osteoporosis because it hastens bone loss.

Benefits Of Milk Overrated

The dairy industry paints an illusory picture of how good milk is for you. In reality, calcium from milk is not readily absorbed because milk's ratio of phosphorus to calcium is 25 to 1. In bones, the ratio is one part phosphorus to two and a half parts calcium. Therefore, the calcium is not readily absorbed. The Vitamin D added to milk for increased calcium absorption is synthetic and is not as effective in metabolizing calcium as natural Vitamin D.

Benefits Of Vitamin K Overlooked

Vitamin K aids in the retention of calcium by reducing the amount excreted in the urine up to 50 percent.

Animals Don't Have A Milkman

It is best to obtain calcium from the same sources the animals do—green leafy vegetables.

Better Treatment For Herniated Disc

Percutaneous discotectomy is a procedure that takes the place of a laminectomy for treating a herniated disc. This innovative method aspirates the protruding part of the disc, releasing pressure on the nerves. It is less traumatic and more cost-effective than debilitating back surgery.

Body Seeks Balance

When the body is in an acid state (during illness), calcium is excreted from the bones to balance blood levels and bring them to a more alkaline level.

Cortisone Makes Mush Of Bones

Cortisone is injected into joints to reduce inflammation. If too much is used, it can cause softening of the bone.

Tennis Elbow

Acupuncture is an effective treatment for tennis elbow.

Bone Loss

A side effect of cortisone is bone loss which occurs by preventing the absorption of protein into the bone. Ingesting too much sugar also causes cortisol levels (cortisone) to rise, leading to osteoporosis.

Building Bone

Calcium has never been proven to build bone mass. It just slows down its decline. Magnesium has been shown to build bone mass. Vitamin K is also needed for production of a certain protein (osteocalsin) in the bone tissue. This protein helps calcium get absorbed from the blood into the bone and allows it to crystallize. Without Vitamin K, this does not happen. Foods containing the most Vitamin K are kelp, alfalfa and leafy greens.

Best Time To Take Calcium

Calcium taken at night is more effective, because remineralization and bone growth take place at night.

Diagnosing Back Pain

Only one percent of people with back pain require surgery. The best diagnostic test for lower back problems is an MRI, since X-rays do not show discs or soft tissue.

Sit Correctly

In a sitting position, most pressure is placed on the lower back. When sitting, keep knees higher than the waist and get up and walk around every 30 minutes.

Sit-Ups

To avoid injuring the lower back, keep knees bent while doing sit-ups.

Beware Of Phosphorus

One reason the body loses calcium is the overingestion of phosphorus which is found in animal-type protein and soft drinks. Phosphorus bonds with calcium and prevents the calcium from being absorbed by the body.

Don't Stop Exercising

After age 30, people who do not maintain an exercise program lose 10 percent of their lean body muscle mass every decade.

Leg Cramps

When leg cramps occur in the calves upon awakening, try performing wall stretches. Stand at arm's length from the wall, with hands braced on the wall and push hard against it.

Back Off From Back Surgery

Asymptomatic people were randomly given MRI's to test for problems. The results showed:

- 52 percent had a bulging disc.
- 22 percent had a bulging protrusion.
- 1 percent had a bulging extrusion.
- 38 percent had an abnormality of one intervertebral disc.

Conclusion—Many people without back pain have disc bulges or protrusions.

Knee Exercise

Walking backwards is one of the best exercises for knee problems.

Sweet Bone Thieves

Too much sugar causes high excretion of calcium from the bones.

Water Cure

Stiffness in older people could be due to dehydration of the joints. Dry joints become brittle and the older person's body has less elasticity. To alleviate this condition, consume eight to ten glasses of liquid (preferably water) daily.

The Best Bike

People with bad knees and bad backs should use a recumbent bicycle where the seat is more like a chair with back support instead of the common non-supporting bicycle seat. The legs of a recumbent bike are on a more horizontal plane which takes the strain off the back and knees.

Sunshine And Fractures

More fractures occur in the winter, not necessarily from falling on the ice, but because of the lack of Vitamin D derived from sunshine. Vitamin D enhances bone growth.

Myelogram

A side effect of a myelogram (injection of a dye into the spinal canal for diagnostic purposes) is a condition known as arachnoiditis, a painful inflammatory condition.

Unfortunately there is no holistic alternative to a myelogram that can visualize the interior area of the spinal column. The patient has to determine if this possible side effect is worth diagnosing a narrowing of the canal.

Running Down Your Spine

People who run more than 40 miles a week may develop less sturdy spines. This could cause shrinkage of overall height and a 10 percent shrinkage of the spine.

Failure Of Spinal Fusions

Spinal fusions do not work in most cases because the bones do not knit properly, due to poor absorption of the minerals needed for continuation of new bone growth. The original bad back is caused by the same process, poor absorption of nutrients.

34 Skin

Acne Rosacea

Spicy foods exacerbate the condition of acne rosacea, a chronic skin disease characterized by redness of the skin tissues and pustules on the face.

Vitiligo

Vitiligo (a skin condition in which smooth white patches form on various parts of the body due to the loss of natural pigment) is caused by the white blood cells attacking the pigment-producing cells in the skin (an autoimmune process). The condition may be related to a deficiency of copper.

Pigment Cell Transplant

If you do have vitiligo, you can have pigment cells transplanted from the parts of your body that manufacture melanin, the pigment that causes skin color.

Don't Suffocate Eczema

Do not use petroleum jelly on eczema. It forms a seal where it is applied and stops oxygen from coming in contact with the inflamed tissue which slows down the healing process.

Go To The Holy Land

Vitamin D helps in the treatment of psoriasis. Sunlight generates Vitamin D production in the skin. Salt water baths are also effective. Many psoriasis sufferers have found relief in the Dead

Sea area of Israel due to the combined effect of the sun and the high concentrate of salt in the water.

Keloids

Keloids are an overgrowth of connective tissue at the site of an incision and they cause ropelike scars. They result from a lack of factor 13 in the blood, and are more prevalent among the black population because of overproliferation of collagen in their skin during the healing process.

Season Your Keloid

Ginger root applied directly to the affected area will help reduce the size of the keloids. Sulfur in the ginger root stimulates chemical activity to help remodel the scar tissue collagen into a more permanent and effective type.

The ABCD's Of Danger Signs In Moles

A—Asymmetry
B—Borders are irregular
C—Change in color
D—Diameter greater than a pencil eraser

Most Dangerous Moles

The most dangerous moles on the body are those located on the back of the legs.

Inside Out

Skin conditions such as seborrhea, psoriasis, eczema, atopical dermatitis and acne rosacea are often related to a systemic yeast infection. This condition can be relieved by eating a high protein, low carbohydrate diet and excluding all sugar, dairy, yeast products (bread, rolls, bagels) and fermented foods (wine, beer, tofu and vinegar).

Go Natural

Use Vitamin A for skin conditions instead of Acutane and Retin A which are merely *derived* from Vitamin A. Acutane can raise cholesterol.

Dry Skin Factors

Vegetarians and those with low cholesterol often have overly dry skin since their diets do not provide the essential fats needed to maintain and facilitate the production of oil in the skin.

Causes Of Skin Conditions

Skin conditions such as acne, seborrhea, psoriasis, eczema, atopical dermatitis, dandruff and fungal infections are usually caused by:

- Allergies
- Blood sugar imbalances
- Deficient autoimmune system
- Nutritional deficiencies
- Yeast infections

Alleviate Acne

Tea tree oil and zinc oxide applied topically are both effective in treating acne. It is important to avoid shellfish, kelp, and supplements containing iodine, since iodine exacerbates acne.

Skin/Colon Connection

Acne is caused by an overload of toxins in the body, in many cases due to constipation. These toxins are released through the skin.

Look At Your Nails

Pulmonary problems cause club nails (convex appearance). Kidney problems cause spoon nails (concave appearance).

Don't Be Thin-Skinned

Steroid creams have a skin-thinning effect which could cause aging of the skin.

Ultraviolet Rays

Ultraviolet rays A and B (UVA and UVB) are the rays that penetrate the atmosphere and cause skin damage.

UVA rays tend to penetrate the skin more deeply and are the ones responsible for aging.

UVB rays cause skin cancer in humans.

Basal cell cancer affects one in six fair-skinned individuals.

Squamous cell cancer occurs one-sixth as often as basal cell cancer.

Malignant melanoma is the most serious.

Sunscreens

Sunscreens should be applied 30 minutes before exposure as they take that long to be absorbed and become effective.

Sunscreens should protect against both UVA and UVB rays. Tanning salons use UVA which can cause skin cancer. A tan is not healthy, it is a sign of injury.

Fluorescent Lights Kill

People who work in areas with fluorescent lighting have a higher rate of melanoma than people who spend hours at the beach in the sun.

Hives

Patients with hives should be tested for helicobacter pylori, the bacteria found to cause stomach ulcers. Hives are sometimes a reaction to this bacteria, rather than an allergen.

Insect Repellant

DEET is an effective insect repellant, but it is toxic to the system when absorbed through the skin and should be sprayed only on outer clothing. Make your own insect repellant by combining:

1/2 ounce citronella

1/4 ounce lavender

1/8 ounce each pennyroyal, eucalyptus, jojoba and tea tree oil in a base of 16 ounces of almond oil.

Ban The Bugs

Brewer's yeast taken internally can ward off insect bites. Topical application of pennyroyal can also be effective.

Don't Be Too Sweet

People who consume high amounts of sugar and carbohydrates tend to get more mosquito bites since their skin exudes a sweetness that attracts insects.

Bee Stings

Household ammonia is an effective remedy for bee stings.

Don't Leave Home Without It

If you are allergic to bee stings, carry an Epi Pen. This is a syringe containing epinephrine in a handy fountain-pen-type applicator. Self-injection with this device could save your life.

Beat The Bite

To alleviate swelling of insect bites, mix three teaspoons of charcoal powder with one teaspoon of slippery elm powder and enough water to form a paste. Apply to bite area.

Test The Tic

If bitten by a tic, save the tic so it can be tested to see if it carries Lyme disease. It is essential to start treatment as soon as possible if you have been bitten by an infected tic. However, there is no point taking antibiotics if the tic is innocuous.

Tic Killer

Tea tree oil kills tics on contact.

Sesame Oil Massage

A warm sesame oil massage will relieve psoriasis lesions.

Skin Tags

Skin tags can be self-treated. Tie a piece of nylon thread tightly around the base and the skin tag will fall off by itself.

Sweeten Your Wound

A wound that is not healing will often respond to ginger and raw honey, which are natural antibiotics.

Scleraderma

High doses of PABA (12 grams daily) act as an anti-fibrous agent and help treat scleraderma.

Warning! Check Your Color

Excessive iron in the system could cause a bronze appearance of the skin.

Rub Warts Away

To get rid of warts, rub them twice daily with the inner part of a banana skin. Also, cut the stem of a dandelion plant and apply the sap.

Act On Acne

Application of tea tree oil to the skin helps alleviate acne eruptions.

Supplements of Vitamin A and zinc enhance the protective factors of the skin.

Shellfish and sea vegetables are high in iodine and should be eliminated from the diet because iodine increases the severity of acne.

Fountain Of Youth

In order to retain a youthful appearance, the body must maintain its ability to eliminate dead skin. Two relatively new methods of accomplishing this are alpha hydroxy acid and Retin A. Here's how they work.

Alpha hydroxy acid stimulates the exfoliation process and washes away the dead cells.

Retin A works by causing the skin to produce more collagen making it plumper and more youthful looking.

Helpful supplements for stimulating collagen production are Vitamin C, cod liver oil and any type of cartilage supplement.

Acne Breakthrough

One cause of acne is an overabundance of oil in the system. This makes intestinal matter back up and produces toxins that are eventually eliminated through the skin. Therefore, intestinal cleansing should be incorporated in the treatment of acne by means of herbs like echinacea, goldenseal, slippery elm bark or American saffron and high fiber.

35 Sleep-Related Problems

Sleep Through The Night

When sleep disorder centers take patients' histories, they never ask for any information regarding their diets. Yet, low blood sugar (hypoglycemia) can lead to such severe disturbances in sleep patterns that the person affected regularly awakens from a deep sleep.

Snoring Can Be A Danger Signal

Sleep apnea (a sudden loss of breathing during sleep) could be either a disturbance of the brain signals that activate breathing or an obstruction that closes the airways. Both could lead to heart problems during sleep due to a lack of oxygen and anyone who has sleep apnea should be evaluated at a sleep disorder center. This disorder is usually discovered by a bed partner, and those who sleep alone may be unaware of the problem. Loud snoring generally precedes sleep apnea, and if you have severe headaches in the morning, they could be caused by this condition.

Alleviate Snoring

An unpleasant aftereffect of the surgery that is done to alleviate snoring (trimming of the uvula) is that liquids tend to back up into the nose when you swallow them. And further, the procedure costs $3,000.00 and is usually not covered by insurance.

Two simpler and cheaper methods to alleviate snoring are:

Losing weight.

Wearing a cervical collar while sleeping.

Thick Neck

Men whose neck size is over 17 inches snore more and have higher rates of sleep apnea. To alleviate this condition, they can use a dental retaining device which stops the tongue from closing off the airway.

Anti-Snoring Device

Breathe Right, an apparatus designed to keep nasal passages open in athletes, also helps eliminate snoring.

Natural Sleep Aids

Dairy products are a good natural source of the amino acid tryptophan which helps you sleep. Or take 8 ounces of pumpkin seeds which produce 1200 mg of tryptophan. Other foods with high amounts of tryptophan are cottage cheese, turkey and avocados.

Benefits Of Melatonin

Melatonin works by controlling the release of adrenalin from the adrenal glands. If too much adrenalin is released while sleeping, then sleep patterns will be disturbed. Another benefit of melatonin is that it aids in the production of serotonin, a mood enhancer. Melatonin also works as an oncostatic agent, protecting the body against cancer.

Sweet Dreams

The herb, Kava Kava, from the root of the pepper plant is an effective substance for relaxation and can be used for insomnia.

Be Negative

Place a negative magnet pole on the forehead to relax. Negative pole magnets are available from:

Dr. Philpot
405-390-3009.

A Good Night's Sleep

Patients with heart disease often have trouble sleeping because their sympathetic nervous system produces too much adrenalin. Adrenalin production should be decreased during sleep and this can be accomplished by using melatonin. Note: Melatonin levels are five times lower in heart patients. Melatonin is also a highly effective free radical scavenger and can be used as an antioxidant. It can be purchased in any health food store.

Narcolepsy

Narcolepsy is a disorder where a person drops off to sleep without warning at inappropriate times. One cause of this phenomenon is low growth hormone levels. These hormones cannot be released unless sleep stages of three or four are reached. These sleep stages occur in the first 3 hours of sleep.

A natural growth hormone releaser is the amino acid L-Arginine, taken in large amounts. This is contraindicated in diabetic patients, especially if they are using insulin. Growth hormone slows the production of insulin. Since Arginine depletes Lysine, it may also exacerbate herpes outbreaks.

36 Smoking And Tobacco-Related Problems

Tobacco Companies Lie

The tobacco companies insist that smoking is not addictive. If so, how come smokers can't quit?

Double Standard

Nicotine patches or nicotine chewing gum are prescription items. But cigarettes, which contain *much* more nicotine, can be purchased anywhere.

More Dangerous Than Russian Roulette

Nicotine is an alkaloid. 60 mg will kill you. Each cigarette produces 2.5 mg of nicotine.

Sweet Death

Some cigarettes are laced with sugar to give them a sweeter taste.

Tobacco Companies Mislead Public

Low tar, low nicotine cigarettes lead to an increase in smoking because smokers need more of them to satisfy their addiction. This leads to even higher sales for the tobacco companies.

Keep Coughing

When giving up smoking it is natural and beneficial to cough to rid the body of accumulated poisons. Do not take cough suppressants as they would only defeat the purpose of this natural process.

Passive Smoking Kills

The risk of lung cancer in non-smoking women increases 80 percent if they live in households with one or more heavy smoker.

Another Reason Not To Smoke

Smoking can also cause bladder cancer.

High Cost Of Smoking

$ 100 billion yearly: Cost to the United States from the ill effects of smoking.

$6,000: The additional amount spent for medical expenses by each smoker during their lifetime.

6.5 days a year: The number of days more that smokers miss work over non-smokers.

6 times more: The number of additional visits per year that smokers make to health practitioners over non-smokers.

$8.6 billion: The cost of lost productivity due to *passive* smoking.

2,300: The number of men, women and children who burn to death in fires caused by cigarettes.

187,000: The number of fires caused yearly by smoking, in the USA alone.

$552,000: The dollar amount of property damage from fires caused by smoking.

$50 billion: The annual sales of a major cigarette manufacturer.

$2 billion: The amount spent for cigarette advertisements and promotional events in 1989.

$3.9 billion: The amount spent for cigarette advertisements and promotional events in 1990.

80: The percentage of six and a half year olds who associate a picture of Old Joe Camel with a package of cigarettes.

$476,000: The amount spent on one brand of cigarettes by smokers under age 18.

56 billion: The number of cigarettes exported in 1984.

194 billion: The number of cigarettes exported by the United States in 1991.

$2.5 million: The amount contributed by the tobacco industry to the Presidential campaign in 1992.

37 Steroids' Side Effects

Hunks Fooled

Ninety-five percent of anabolic steroids being used by athletes are fake.

Teenagers Looking For Trouble

Ten percent of high school athletes use anabolic steroids. These lower the good cholesterol (HDL) and can also cause cancer.

Lost Muscle Gain

As soon as you stop taking steroids, the muscle mass that was gained is rapidly lost.

Bodybuilders Beware

Anabolic steroids can build muscle mass more quickly. They are body nutrients that activate the protein building system and enhance healing. However, their negative effects far outweigh the positive ones. They can cause aggression, negative effects on the reproductive system, liver tumors, high blood pressure and heart disease. These side effects may not be immediately apparent, but occur later in life.

38 Thyroid

Synthroid Enhancer

Patients taking synthroid, a thyroid-stimulating hormone, will not get the full effect unless their systems have adequate amounts of Vitamin B^6, selenium and zinc to get the synthroid into an active state.

Synthetic Substitutes

Patients who don't respond to synthroid (thyroid replacement hormone) should try Armour thyroid, which is natural desiccated animal thyroid. It has no side effects and also has the advantage of containing calcitonin which protects the body from calcium and bone loss.

Natural Vs Synthetic

Armour thyroid (natural extract of animal gland) has T3 and T4 and calcitonin. Synthroid has only T4. The T4 should convert into T3, but in certain cases this does not happen.

No Symptoms—No Synthroid

If a routine blood test shows high TSH (indicating an underactive thyroid) but the T4 is normal, it is an indication that the thyroid is adequately compensating for its low production of thyroxin. Without the accompanying symptoms of low thyroid such as cold hands, dry skin, hair loss, tiredness, weight gain and constipation, do not allow your practitioner to automatically prescribe synthroid.

Sustained Release Thyroid

Thyroid medication should be administered in a sustained release form in order to more nearly mimic the body's biological output of thyroid hormone.

Dangerous Water

Chlorine and fluoride in water are enzyme blockers. They are also halogens which block the iodine needed for the thyroid to function properly. Boiling the water removes only the chlorine, not the fluoride.

Body Temperature

Thyroid function should be checked in people with allergies. Even if blood thyroid levels are normal, a dysfunction could be present. This can be checked by taking your body temperature orally. If it is below 97.6, that could mean you have hypothyroidism (an underactive thyroid). And hypothyroidism can be the underlying factor in many diseases, including cancer. Viruses and bacteria live longer in a body with a lower temperature. A higher body temperature tends to destroy viruses and bacteria because fever is the body's natural defense against these invaders.

Thyroid Medication Administration

To be most effective, thyroid medication should be taken with the same food at the same time of day.

Better Testing For Thyroid

If T.S.H. tests results for underactive or overactive thyroid are not conclusive, the more accurate diagnostic Thyroid Releasing Hormone Test (an injection), should be utilized.

Thyroid And Bowel Function

Thyroid function affects bowel function. Low thyroid function causes constant constipation, and an overactive (high) thyroid often leads to loose bowels and diarrhea.

Hyperthyroidism

Graves disease (Hyperthyroidism) may burn itself out completely in a few years.

Keep Levels Up

Progesterone facilitates thyroid function. Progesterone levels drop drastically as females enter menopause. This can lead to hypothyroidism and a resulting weight gain. Progest cream ameliorates this condition.

Don't Table The Salt

A low salt diet causes thyroid malfunction since iodized salt is a prime source of iodine in the American Diet. The establishment's dietary advice to patients with high blood pressure has been to reduce salt intake. Since the American way of thinking is to overdo advice, if a suggestion is made to cut down on something, they will tend to cut it out entirely.

The thyroid gland needs iodine to function properly. Patients who cut out iodized salt should take supplements containing iodine or increase their intake of sea vegetables (kelp) and shellfish.

Chlorine And Fluoride

The chlorine and fluoride found in most municipal water supplies block iodine receptors in the thyroid gland (they are chemically related to iodine) and this can eventually lead to hypothyroidism. It is also important to check your toothpaste as many brands contain fluoride.

39 TMJ—Temporomandibular Joint

The Often Overlooked Malady

Clenching or grinding the teeth while sleeping is often caused by temporomandibular joint misalignment.

Headaches and tic douloureux (a severe facial neuralgia accompanied by convulsive twitching of the facial muscles) can be caused by temporomandibular joint misalignment.

Clenching Self-Check

Set a timer for every 20 minutes while you're awake, to remind you to check if you are clenching your teeth.

Tinnitus? Check Your Jaw

A misaligned temporomandibular joint (TMJ) could be a possible cause of tinnitus.

40 Ulcers

Cayenne

Cayenne is a universal treatment for ulcers. Its healing power has been known for years and it is used everywhere except in the United States.

Slippery Elm

Slippery elm bark soothes ulcers and stomach upset and destroys the bacteria (campylobacter) that causes ulcers.

Deglycyrrhizinated Licorice

Deglycyrrhizinated licorice is the only substance in the entire history of mankind to have a curative effect on ulcers.

Pepto-Bismol And Ulcers

Pepto-Bismol inhibits the campylobacter bacteria (the bacteria that causes ulcers). It contains bismuth.

Metallic Taste

A constant metallic taste in the mouth could be caused by a bacteria which lives in the lining of the stomach (helicobacter pylori). Individuals with type O blood are more prone to H.B.P. A simple blood test can determine this.

41 Yeast (Candida)

Safe Yeast Treatment

Nystatin is one of the few drugs that are safe, because it is not absorbed by the system but goes directly to the site of the Candida.

Medication Warning

Many doctors are now prescribing Nizoral instead of Nystatin to treat fungal infections. Be sure not to take Nizoral if you are taking the new antihistamines that cause less drowsiness such as Seldane. The combination is extremely dangerous and could lead to death.

Itchy Anus

An itchy anus may be due to a yeast problem. This condition can be relieved by eating a high protein, low carbohydrate diet and excluding all sugar, dairy, yeast products (bread, rolls, bagels) and fermented foods (wine, beer, tofu and vinegar).

Accurate Diagnosis Of Candida

To get an accurate diagnosis of Candida, it is necessary to check blood levels for antibodies against Candida and also check the stool for antibodies and parasites. Most physicians do not test the stool.

Candida Exacerbators

Progesterone or cortisone inflame a Candida problem.

Complete Candida Treatment

Treatment for Candida should also include treatment for parasites which are also present when this condition exists.

Thorough Candida Stool Test

Yeast lives in the feces. Parasites live in the feces and also on the lining of the colon. A stool sample doesn't necessarily show the presence of parasites because, by the time the stool is analyzed in the laboratory (often two to three days after taking the sample), most of them have disappeared. For a proper diagnosis, the colon should be swabbed to pick up the live parasites, and the sample should be immediately analyzed under the microscope. Most orthodox doctors do not swab the colon.

Don't Feed The Parasites

If parasites are present, avoid therapeutic juicing from fruit. Green juicing is allowable.

Hasten Digestion

If transit time of food consumed takes more than 18 hours, an overgrowth of abnormal pathogenic material (parasites and yeast) may occur. Ascorbic C and glutathione shorten the transit time.

One Thing Leads To Another

A common side effect of flagyl (medication used to treat parasites) is the growth of too much yeast.

Symptoms Of Yeast Infection

- Athlete's foot
- Bloating
- Fatigue
- Frequent touching of genitals
- Memory loss
- Nail fungus
- Red ring around the anus
- Smelly feet
- White tongue

Yeast In Stomach

Antacids and/or Tagamet can exacerbate an existing yeast infection in the stomach.

Unrecognized Danger

Orthodox practitioners treat only symptoms of a systemic yeast infestation, disregarding the fact that it is an ongoing disease. Candida is caused by a lack of oxygen in the cells, and the same deficiencies that cause it can also lead to cancer.

Check For Diabetes

Women who get repeated vaginal infections should be checked for diabetes since the vaginal area of diabetics is more conductive to the growth of yeast.

Get Shot

If a severe bacterial infection requires antibiotic therapy, have the antibiotics administered by injection rather than orally to avoid having them pass through the intestinal tract. This will help to avoid gastrointestinal problems, such as diarrhea.

42 Miscellaneous

Snakebite

In cases of snakebite, it is urgent to treat the victim for shock because the foreign protein in the venom causes shock, killing the patient.

Heating System

Homes with forced hot air heating systems can be drier than the Sahara Desert. Use a humidifier, especially at night in the bedroom.

Oxygen Levels

Mucous in the body indicates that oxygen levels are low in the cells. To oxidize the body, use ozone or hydrogen peroxide (35% grade). Ozone therapy is administered intravenously or by insulfation (through the rectum).

Botulism

Botulism kills by paralyzing the intestinal muscles.

Powerful Antibiotic

Oxygen is the most powerful antibiotic and kills parasites.

Ozone

The broadest (most effective) antibiotic known to man is ozone, and it has no side effects. The cells, through a process of free radical destruction, convert from the aerobic form (with oxygen) to the anaerobic form (without oxygen). This causes a proliferation of viruses and bacteria which cannot live in an aerobic environment. Ozone therapy is a process of adding an extra molecule of oxygen to the blood supply. The extra molecule of oxygen, derived from hydrogen peroxide (H_20_2), causes the destruction of the viruses and bacteria.

Protect Your Voice

Singers and speakers should be aware of the following facts.

1. Acid can rise up from the stomach and irritate the larynx (voice box).

2. Ninety percent of any nodules on the vocal cords will disappear spontaneously. Surgery on nodules causes scar tissue which could destroy the voice.

3. Nose jobs (plastic surgery) or reconstructive dental work can change the quality of the voice.

What The White Count Shows

A low white blood count can be a sign of a viral infection. A high white blood count usually indicates a bacterial infection.

Night Sweats

Night sweats could be caused by tuberculosis. TB medication has terrible side effects, including liver damage, impotence, headaches and elevated blood sugar levels. Use Vitamin B^6 to counteract the side effects.

Improper Breathing

If you do not breathe properly, sighing is often an attempt to inhale more oxygen. Improper breathing can lead to poor elimination of carbon dioxide, causing the blood to become more acid and, if blood is too acidic, the cells will become dysfunctional.

Ladybug Ladybug Fly To My Home

Instead of using toxic chemicals which cause disease, use ladybugs to effectively control insects on plants.

Excess Iron

If you have excess iron in your system, you should donate blood three times a year. Chelation therapy will also remove too much iron from the system.

TIA—Mini Stroke

TIA, transient ischemic attack, is usually followed by a stroke in two years.

Oxidants

Copper and iron have an oxidant effect on the system opposite to antioxidant. Oxidants cause free radicals which lead to the breakdown of normal cell function and subsequent disease.

Our Miraculous Bodies

The human body has nine times the amount of liver needed for survival. The liver regenerates every six weeks.

You can survive with as little as one-tenth of your liver intact.

A person can survive on one-quarter of one healthy kidney and one-quarter of a stomach.

The bones rebuild every three months.

The stomach lining changes every five days.

The skin is renewed every month.

Night Sweats

Night sweats may be a symptom of tuberculosis or Hodgkin's disease.

Cold Baths

Cold water baths have the following beneficial effects. They:

- Are an antidote to depression.
- Boost the immune system.
- Can slow the aging process.
- Increase testosterone levels in men.
- Relieve asthma attacks.

Lyme Disease

Colostrum from cows injected with the dead Lyme virus is useful in the treatment of Lyme disease.

Best Aerobic Exercise

The most effective aerobic exercise is cross-country skiing.

Chronic Fatigue

Chronic fatigue sufferers should have their adrenal glands checked, especially if they have low blood pressure. Use deglycrrhizinated licorice to strengthen adrenal function and raise blood pressure.

Quick Absorption Method

The fastest and most effective way to get a substance into the bloodstream is to smoke it.

Scans Can't See Everything

Small lesions of less than one millimeter will not be picked up by an MRI or a CAT scan.

Seat Belts In Buses And Taxis

Be sure to wear a seat belt in the back of a taxi because a sudden stop can throw you against the divider between the front and back seats and cause severe facial or head injuries. Most buses are not equipped with seat belts, and you should never sit directly behind the driver if a divider is present.

Zap Chlorine

Safer, more effective, alternative methods are available for all the major uses of chlorine.

1. Grow food without chlorinated pesticides using organic farming methods. The United States National Research Council has said these are actually more effective and cost-efficient than inorganic methods, and increase the yield besides.

2. Dry clean clothes using a steam and water-based process instead of one using toxic solvents.

3. Manufacture paper using oxygen-based bleaching methods.

4. Disinfect drinking water and swimming pools with sand filtration, ultraviolet light or ozone treatment.

Chlorine Control

Even though you have a filter on your drinking water, chlorine is still absorbed by the body in the shower and the swimming pool. Since it goes directly into the system through the eyes and mouth, it is essential to wear protective goggles while swimming and to keep the mouth closed while showering. Flushing a toilet also releases chlorine into the air. Be sure to close the lid when flushing.

Ceramic filters are more effective for tap water than carbon filters. Carbon filters remove pathogens only down to one micron, and parasites are smaller so they can penetrate this. Ceramic filters can remove pathogens down to 0.5 microns, and that is small enough to stop parasites.

Dry Cleaning Is A Health Hazard

Trichlorethyline, used for dry cleaning, is hazardous to health. Be sure to air clothes thoroughly before storing them in the bedroom closet.

Healthier Buildings In Sweden

Construction materials in Sweden are non-toxic, thereby eliminating sick building syndrome.

The Right Kind Of Light

Exposure to standard house light (in contrast to full spectrum light) tends to clump blood cells and slow blood circulation. As soon as one is exposed to full spectrum light, the clumping starts to break up and circulation begins to normalize. Light *should* be considered a nutrient with an RDA.

Tired? Raise Your Body Temperature

If your body temperature is one degree below normal, you lose 20 to 25 percent of your manufactured body energy.

Acupuncture Signals

Acupuncture signals the brain to direct healing energy to a particular spot.

Always Tired?

Chronic fatigue can be caused by:

- Anemia
- Chemical allergies (perfume, carpets, detergents, paint)
- Low thyroid
- Medications
- Metabolic abnormalities (sugar metabolism)
- Multiple food allergies
- Parasites
- Stress
- Yeast infections

Detox In Your Bathtub

Soak for 20 minutes in a tub of warm water to which 12 ounces of food grade hydrogen peroxide has been added (available in health food stores, this is not the three and a half percent used for antiseptic purposes). This aids in the detoxification of poisonous elements and viruses including cancer, AIDS and hepatitis.

Genetics Is Not A Death Sentence

Genetics is not a destiny. It is a predisposition. A family history of a disease does not always mean a person will contract that disease. Lifestyle changes, enhanced diet, added supplements, exercise and a positive attitude can fortify the immune system so effectively that the "inevitable" can be staved off.

Lymphatic Cleansing

A lymphatic cleansing device, originally used to reduce swelling in the arm following axillary node removal, has also been proven effective for other conditions resulting from thickened blood, such as poor circulation, thrombosis, varicose veins and coronary artery disease. It works by changing positively-charged cells to negatively-charged ones that repel each other.

This prevents clotting and allows freer blood flow. It is called the Particle Beam Generator Lymphotec Machine.

Toxic Environment

70,000 chemicals that are potentially neurotoxic exist in the environment. Of these, only five percent have been tested for neurotoxicity. The most common is dioxin, in the form of a chlorine bleaching process found in most paper goods. Try to buy unbleached toilet paper, paper towels, coffee filters and napkins.

Polio Vaccine

Every case of polio since 1979 has been caused by the polio vaccine, according to information from the Centers for Disease Control. Ninety percent of the population exposed to the polio virus will not contract the disease.

Tonsils

Tonsils shrink as one grows older. They involute.

Test For Adrenal Function

To test adrenal function, take your blood pressure in a sitting position. Wait one minute, then take a standing blood pressure reading. The standing reading should be 10 percent higher. If not, adrenal function is inadequate.

Body Sculpting

It is safer for individuals to use their *own* fat for body sculpting, instead of using collagen or silicone.

Charge It

The normal human body has a negative charge. Bacteria, viruses and pathogens carry a positive charge.

Flooding the body with oxygen or ozone introduces negatively-charged particles which scavenge and rout all positively-charged elements harmful to the body.

Acupuncture Beats The Patch

The scopalamine patch used for seasickness and motion sickness can cause sleepiness and dry mouth. Acupressure wrist bands are more effective for this and have no side effects.

Uric Acid A Barometer For Disease

High amounts of uric acid can cause gout. Uric acid is a natural antioxidant. If the levels are too low, it can mean the body is fighting too many free radicals with too suppressed an immune system.

Iron Deficiency

People with a craving to chew ice cubes are iron deficient.

Stinky Feet

To alleviate smelly feet, wash them with alcohol.

Old Fashioned Remedy

Epsom salts baths are effective because the magnesium in the salts is absorbed through the skin into the system, and magnesium is a relaxant.

Bugs Resist Antibiotics

The response rate to medically-prescribed antibiotics has decreased dramatically. In 1941, pneumonia could be cured with 41,000 units of penicillin. Today, it takes 24 million units. The reason for this is the microbes have mutated and developed a protective mechanism against antibiotics.

Drug Addiction

An effective alternative method for treating drug addiction is acupuncture. This is being done with good results at Lincoln Hospital in the Bronx, New York.

Deadly Sport

More fatal accidents are caused by horseback riding than any other sport, including boxing.

Killer Drugs

Diuretics also cause the loss of magnesium, an integral electrolyte needed for electrolyte balancing.

Cholesterol-lowering drugs cause the loss of Co-Enzyme Q-10, an enzyme that is essential for the cell's energy production.

The package insert for Lopressor contains four separate warnings about its harmful effects on the heart. One of them specifically states that this drug may bring on a heart attack.

Side Effect Of Flu Shot

More people get sick from the side effects of a flu shot than from the flu itself.

Part III

- *Food And Beverages*
- *Supplements*
- *Uses Of Herbs*

43 Food And Beverages

MEAT

Beware The Barbecue

As meat is cooked, fat drips onto the flame, combines with hydrocarbons in the flame, then rises into the cooked meat. This leads to the production of carcinogenic molecules which can cause cancer when the meat is consumed.

Desirable Animal Parts

Eat the parts of the animal that move, such as the shoulder and rump, rather than the glands and organs where the toxins accumulate.

Wild Birds And Game

Wild birds and animals have only three to four percent body fat since their diet consists of grasses, berries and leaves. Farm animals are fed corn and soy products and are inundated with hormones. Therefore it is healthier to eat game such as venison, buffalo, rabbit, partridge and pheasant, which also contain higher levels of the essential fatty acids needed to prevent inflammation in the body.

Antibiotics In Our Food Supply

Fifty percent of all antibiotics produced in the United States are given to animals used for food. Therefore, people are ingesting antibiotics unknowingly.

Farm animals and poultry are given antibiotics constantly, not just when needed for fighting infections. This is done to insure that the animals will not contract any disease that will make them lose weight. People who consume this meat and poultry are constantly ingesting antibiotics and this eventually makes their bodies resistant to the medical antibiotics they may need to treat diseases.

Europeans Nix U.S. Meat

Importation of meat from the United States is frowned on in Europe because of our use of hormones and antibiotics.

Organic Meats Safer

Organic meats contain 30 percent less fat because the animals are not given hormones to fatten them. Chemicals tend to collect in the fatty tissues, and the fat of non-organic meats contains large amounts of hormones and antibiotics.

Bad Burgers

Fecal matter has been found in 30 percent of all ground beef and children have died because of this contamination.

Pork Vs Beef

Pork is lower in saturated fat than beef.

FISH AND SEAFOOD

Eat Fish—Live Longer

The Japanese eat five to seven times more fish than the Americans and they live five to seven years longer, with less cancer and fewer heart problems.

Don't Microwave Fish

Fish cooked in a microwave releases 20 times as much mercury as fish cooked by conventional methods. Released mercury damages the system while unreleased mercury is not absorbed.

Shellfish

Shellfish are high in cholesterol, but low in fat.

Tuna Fish

Tuna fish is high in selenium.

Seafood

Seafood is rich in selenium, zinc and iodine.

Sushi

Fish used for sushi should be frozen first in order to kill parasites.

Small Fish

Smaller fish are lower in the food chain and contain fewer pollutants.

A Drink May Save Your Life

Some oysters contain a harmful bacteria that can lead to fatal disease. Drinking alcohol while eating oysters helps to kill this bacteria.

Polluted Waters

Eating fish from polluted waters causes genetic changes in people of childbearing age, leading to the danger of physical and mental defects in their offspring.

Dairy Products

Goat's Milk

Goat's milk has less fat than cow's milk because goats are smaller animals and they are not flooded with hormones.

Milk Sensitivities

Children and adults with sensitivities to milk or soy products can drink Nutramagin which contains neither dairy nor soy. Its protein is derived from casein, a milk protein that is enzymatically hydrolyzed (broken down) so that no trace of the allergic milk protein remains.

Bovine Growth Hormone

Dairy cows given BST (bovine growth hormone) have a 70 percent rise in mastitis (inflammation of the udder). This increases the animal's need for antibiotics which eventually get absorbed by milk consumers, especially children. This causes prescribed antibiotics to be less effective in treating bacterial infections.

Almond Milk

Individuals who are sensitive to soy, goat or rice milk may find almond milk more tolerable.

What's In The Milk

The public is told one glass of milk equals 300 mg of calcium and 100 I.U. of Vitamin D. However, the Vitamin D is a synthetic form and the calcium to phosphorus ratio is so out of balance that it is difficult for the body to absorb it. Other unnatural ingredients found in milk are antibiotics, tranquilizers, growth hormone and pesticides.

Butter Is Better

The buteric acid in butter has anti-microbial properties. Buteric acid is a natural healing therapy used for leukemia and colitis.

Clarified Butter

Clarified butter (ghee) does not become rancid and can be stored indefinitely. It is stable because the water and milk solids have been removed. Ghee is available in health food stores.

WATER

Beverages Consumed

Each individual in the United States drinks an average of 187.7 gallons of fluid a year. Only 16 percent of this is pure water. 26 percent of beverages consumed are soft drinks which contain either large amounts of sugar or potentially dangerous levels of artificial sweeteners.

Don't Drink The Water

Environmental studies show that from one-sixth to one-third of the nation's water supplies are contaminated with coliform bacteria (sewage).

Dechlorinate Your Water

An easy, no cost way to get rid of the chlorine in drinking water is to put it in a container and let it sit at least 12 hours.

Distilled Water

Distilled water does not contain any bacteria or viruses.

Water Loss

Adults lose a quart and a half of water daily just from breathing.

Lead Where You Don't Expect It

Tap water is acidic and leaches lead from the solder in the pipes. Counter-type filters do not remove the lead.

Crystal decanters for wine contain lead.

FRUITS AND VEGETABLES

Vegetarians

Vegetarians lack B^{12}, iron, zinc, cholesterol, Vitamin D and essential amino acids in their diets. To avoid malnutrition, it is important for them to consume beans and grains together and take supplements.

Adequate Protein

In order for vegetarians to get adequate protein, they should add tempeh or wheat gluten to their diet.

Buy Organic Produce

Organic produce has twice as many minerals as produce grown with pesticides and chemical fertilizers. It also contains fewer heavy metals such as aluminum, cadmium, lead and mercury.

Quick Digestion

Fruits are the easiest foods to digest, and take only 20 minutes to pass through the stomach and turn into energy. Therefore, if you have low energy, you should consume more fruit in order not to deplete an already weakened system. Vegetables require only slightly more energy to digest. Note: This diet does not apply to diabetics or hypoglycemics.

Apples

One apple equals five grams of fiber.

Artichokes

Artichokes enhance the liver's capacity to detoxify the body by helping it manufacture digestive enzymes and, at the same time, naturally lower cholesterol. Of all foods, artichokes lead the list in aiding digestive problems.

Jerusalem Artichokes

Jerusalem artichokes strengthen the liver's defense against disease.

Natural Diuretic

Asparagus is an effective diuretic.

Avocados

Avocados are rich in Vitamin E and they contain the most fiber of any fruit.

Good Beans

Genestein in soybeans acts like Tamoxifen in the body. It protects the cells from too much estrogen and triggers useful repair enzymes. It also acts as an antiangiogenesis agent (it cuts off the blood supply to tumors).

Broccoli

Eat one cup of broccoli for your daily requirement of folic acid, an important nutrient for treating cervical dysplasia, anemia, colitis and gum disease. Folic acid is depleted by anti-seizure medication.

All About Carrots

- Two carrots a day can reduce cholesterol by 20 percent.
- Carrots are high in calories and sugar content.
- One eight ounce glass of carrot juice contains 200 calories.
- One average carrot contains 48 calories.
- One carrot equals 5000 I.U.'s of beta-carotene.

Citrus Bioflavanoids

Freezing orange or grapefruit juice removes the bioflavanoids necessary to protect the juice from oxidation. Drink fresh-squeezed juice to get those bioflavanoids!

Dandelion Greens

Dandelion greens, ounce for ounce, have as much calcium as dairy products.

Mushrooms

Shiitake mushrooms, or capsules made from them, are natural blood thinners.

Parsley

Parsley thins the blood.

Peanut Butter

Peanut butter is 70 percent fat.

Salsa

Use salsa for a flavorful fat-free dressing.

OIL

All About Oil

Polyunsaturated oils include safflower, sunflower and corn. These stay liquid at room temperature, are not very stable and tend to form free radicals in the system. They become rancid more quickly than saturated fats when they are heated.

Hydrogenated oils are vegetable oils that are solid at room temperature. They are produced in a vacuum. Some nickel is added, and hydrogen gas is pumped in. The body cannot break down this type of oil.

Monounsaturated oils include olive, sesame, canola, peanut and walnut. They are healthier than polyunsaturated oils as they do not turn rancid so quickly.

Saturated oils include coconut and palm and have a higher saturated fat content. They are found in most commercial baked goods and crackers. The body cannot break down these fats. One tablespoon of these oils equals 115 calories.

Altered Oils

Margarine is composed of oils that are natural and healthy, until they are processed with heat, pressure and platinum, a chemical catalyst. Then these once-healthy oils transform into an unnatural state, producing free radicals that lead to disease. These altered oils become trans fatty acids, which raise cholesterol the same as saturated fats.

Cottonseed Oil

Cottonseed oil, found in most bakery items in the supermarket, contains high levels of pesticides from spraying the plants. Yet, despite the fact that pesticides are a known carcinogenic substance, the FDA allows it to be used. For more information on the harmful effects of pesticides, read *The Silent Spring* by Rachael Carson.

What's In A Name

Mazola oil derives its name from maize which means corn.

SWEETS AND SWEETENERS

Sugar Is Not So Sweet

All societies with low sugar ingestion have low rates of heart disease and diabetes. Eskimos, Icelanders, Laplanders and desert nomads fall into this category and retain their health until they relocate into a society with high sugar consumption.

Vanilla Extract

Vanilla extract contains corn syrup.

Calorie Content

One ounce of chocolate contains 147 calories.

One egg contains 50 calories.

Honey

Historically, honey has been the most used therapeutic agent. Bacteria cannot grow in honey and it never spoils. Applied to wounds, it has antibiotic properties. Be sure to use unprocessed certified honey. To soothe a sore throat, gargle with a mixture of honey and lemon juice, then swallow the mixture.

Tingle Your Taste Buds

To eliminate sugar craving, it is critical to stimulate *all* your taste buds daily. The taste sensations are:

Sweet - sugary foods.

Sour - cheese, lemons, yogurt.

Bitter - leafy greens, spinach, endive.

Salty - lox, herring, pickles, anchovies.

Pungent - red pepper, mustard, spices.

Astringent - beans and peas.

If all these sensations are included in your daily diet, your excessive sugar cravings will diminish.

Artificial Sweeteners

Artificial sweeteners can cause seizures, migraines, cardiac arrhythmias and rapid heart rate. The artificial sweeteners MSG and aspartane are first cousins. Aspartane is 10 percent methane, also known as wood alcohol, and known to cause death, seizures, blindness, and possibly increase the size of brain tumors.

Most negative information on aspartane has been suppressed.

Artificial Sweeteners Backfire

People who use artificial sweeteners do not satisfy their sugar craving, and therefore still crave foods with a higher sugar content.

Better Sugar Substitute

Stevia, or glycerine, is a good replacement for sugar.

Candy For Breakfast

Most commercial brands of cereal contain so much sugar that people, especially children, are actually eating candy for breakfast.

Poison In Your Food

DDT

DDT will not be cleared out of the bloodstream in a lifetime. We absorb this chemical through food. DDT causes the thinning of eggshells which leads to deformities of the egg and the chick.

MSG

MSG, monosodium glutamate, exaggerates brain activity and can excite a cell to death. It is present in food enhancers such as hydrolized protein, which consists of 20 percent MSG, and sodium or calcium caseinate (found in certain dairy products) which consists of 12 percent MSG.

Hidden Password

Hydrolized vegetable protein, HVP, is a hidden password for MSG and sodium caseinate.

Interpreting Food Additives

Monosodium phosphate is an emulsifying agent. It has no known toxicity.

Maltodextrin is a flavor enhancer with no known toxicity.

Potassium Bromide is a preservative. It *is* toxic to the central nervous system.

Propylacetate is a flavoring agent for beverages. It is irritating to the skin and the mucous membranes.

Myrrh is a flavoring agent. No known toxicity.

MSG (monosodium glutamate) is a flavor enhancer. It has been known to cause chest pain, headaches and numbness. It may even cause brain damage.

Modified starch modifies thickening or gelling. It is presently listed for re-evaluation by the FDA.

Hydrolyzed vegetable protein is a flavor enhancer. The FDA recommends further study.

Humectants preserve moisture content. No known toxicity.

Gum is an emulsifier, stabilizer and suspending agent. No known toxicity.

Bromate is a maturing agent and dough conditioner. It is *poisonous* to the central nervous system.

Brominated vegetable oils are emulsifying agents in liquids. They are on the suspect list.

Disodium phosphate is an emulsifier. It can irritate skin and mucous membranes.

Invert sugar consists of 50 percent glucose and 50 percent fructose. No known toxicity.

Palmitic acid is a flavoring agent. No known toxicity.

Calcium phosphate is a dough conditioner and firming agent. No known toxicity.

Calcium propionate is a preservative. The FDA recommends further study for safety.

HELPFUL FOODS

Germanitives

Germanitive type foods, such as eggs, nuts, seeds and sprouts, produce more nutrients than any other types of food. Seeds and nuts should be eaten raw. Eggs should be poached or boiled, not fried, since frying the egg in oil or butter exposes it to high temperatures and oxygen, a combination which can produce free radicals (toxic by-products of the combination of oxygen and heat). These free radicals start to break down normal cells which change genetically and then become diseased.

Sources Of B^3

A vitamin B^3 deficiency can lead to the 4 D's: Death, Dermatitis, Diarrhea and Dementia. Food sources of B^3 include beans, vegetables and whole grains.

Sea Salt

Use sea salt rather than processed salt because it does not contain additives, aluminum or bleaching agents.

Protective Foods And Herbs

Citrus fruits protect DNA.

A component of strawberries deactivates cancer-causing molecules and makes them harmless.

Ginger contains oils that help stimulate digestion and alleviate nausea and motion sickness. It is more effective than dramamine.

Curry aids digestion.

Cloves are an effective topical anesthetic.

Cinnamon contains tannin which acts as an astringent and can control diarrhea.

Sage dries up body secretions in the lungs and nasal passages and alleviates sweaty palms.

Cayenne eliminates too much mucous in the lungs.

Ten drops of Tabasco sauce in water, taken 3 or 4 times a day, helps circulation problems and hypertension.

Seeds For Magnesium

Good sources of magnesium are pumpkin seeds, peanut butter and sesame seeds.

Bees

The world's most perfect food is manufactured by bees. Twelve tablets of bee pollen on an empty stomach every half-hour often relieves symptoms of allergies and asthma. Bee propolis is a potent natural antibiotic and royal jelly is a natural energizer.

Red Pepper

Red pepper is the most concentrated source of vitamin C. It can also be used as a blood thinner and stimulant and reduces the pain of ulcerative colitis.

Good Sources Of Selenium

Brazil nuts, fish, eggs, beans and onions all contain high amounts of selenium.

Glutathione

An ingredient found in egg yolks, APO Protein E, is necessary for glutathione, a sulfur-containing amino acid, to activate enzymes that detoxify the liver. Despite the cholesterol craze and all the negative publicity from orthodox physicians and dietitians, two whole eggs should be eaten daily. The best sources of glutathione are raw spinach and parsley.

Rebuild The Liver

Arrowroot powder mixed with licorice root will help rebuild the liver.

Reduce Sweating

Sage tea reduces excessive sweating of feet and night sweats.

Ginger

Ginger warms the body and also relieves muscle pain.

Benefits Of Cayenne

It is a vasodilator (helps keep arteries open).

It cleans clogged arterioles and capillaries.

It increases the blood supply to ulcers and causes a layer of mucous to form over the ulcer, protecting it from stomach acid. The ulcer heals behind this protective shield.

Note: Ginger enhances the absorption of cayenne.

Grapefruit Seed Extract

Grapefruit seed extract is an anti-fungicide. That is why you never see a moldy grapefruit.

Sources Of Bioflavanoids

Bioflavanoids (polyphenols, plant chemicals) help to maintain the integrity of the membrane covering the cell and allow the smooth passage of nutrients from the bloodstream to the cell. The greatest amounts are found in:

- Black tea
- Broccoli
- Celery
- Cranberries
- Endive
- French beans
- Green tea
- Kale
- Onions

Bioflavanoids are also in:

- Apples
- Broad beans
- Grapes
- Lettuce
- Red peppers
- Red wine
- Strawberries
- Tomato juice
- Tomatoes

Stimulate Saliva

Chew on ginger and lemon peel to stimulate the flow of saliva. This helps with dry mouth caused by radiation to the facial area or by medication. Sour foods, such as lemons, oranges, grapes and tomatoes, and the act of chewing also stimulate saliva flow.

Green Tea

Green tea, useful in the treatment and prevention of cancer, contains caffeine. Anyone sensitive to caffeine should drink it early in the day, and people on blood thinners should avoid green tea which is high in Vitamin K, a clotting agent.

Watch Out For

Processed Foods

Foods processed at high temperatures are damaged by the heat and are depleted of their nutrients. Powdered instant mashed potatoes and other types of dehydrated foods have very little nutritional value.

Iron And Copper

Antioxidants (C, E, beta-carotene, selenium and B-complex) reduce the oxidative process which can cause cell destruction. Large amounts of oxidants such as iron and copper cause the oxidation process.

Those with hyperthyroidism and Wilson's Disease should limit their intake of foods containing large amounts of copper. These include liver, whole grains, almonds, green leafy vegetables, dried legumes and sea food.

People who suffer from arthritis and heart conditions should limit their intake of foods with large amounts of iron. These include liver, oysters, lean meat, leafy green vegetables, whole grains, dried fruits, legumes and molasses.

Soy Sauce

Soy sauce is what stimulates the appetite two hours after eating Chinese food.

Pitfall Of Juicing

One pitfall of juicing is that all the fiber is removed. Fiber is necessary for regulation of the bowels.

Pasta

Latest reports show pasta can actually cause weight gain due to the amount consumed. However, the study did not consider the difference between pasta made with white flour vs pasta made with whole wheat flour. Nor did the study take into consideration the high sugar content of tomato sauce.

Poppy Seeds And Drug Tests

Poppy seeds used as a topping on bagels or other baked goods can cause a marijuana test to be positive.

44 Supplements

Vitamin E And Allergies

People who are allergic to wheat or soy should not take natural Vitamin E which is derived from these products. They should use dry Vitamin E rather than the oil form, but they must use twice as much since dry E is only half as potent. E acetate or succinate are synthetic forms of dry Vitamin E.

Nicotine Replacement

Niacin, which is similar in chemical form to nicotine, can be used to help stop smoking because it decreases the craving.

Cranberry Juice Too Sweet

To treat bladder infections, use cranberry extract (a pill) rather than juice which contains too much sugar and further proliferates the negative bacteria leading to even more infection.

Prevent Niacin Flush

To prevent the hot red flush from niacin, take ½ aspirin ½ hour before taking the niacin (B^3).

Diabetic Warning

Don't use niacin if you have diabetes. Niacin raises glucose levels.

Ringing In The Ears

Niacin is useful for treatment of Ménière's disease, a disorder of the inner ear marked by ringing in the ears and some deafness. Niacin is a vasodilator and enhances blood supply to the small capillaries of the inner ear.

Slow Down Calcium Loss

Vitamin K helps fractures heal faster by reducing the amount of calcium excreted in the urine by 50 percent. It is also valuable in treating osteoporosis, lowering blood pressure and getting better sleep.

"D" Transportation System

Vitamin D is needed to transport calcium from the stomach to the bloodstream.

Oil Your Keloid

A keloid is a scar that has overgrown its boundaries and is classified as a benign tumor. The orthodoxy treats keloids with steroid injections. Natural healing therapy utilizes daily application of Vitamin E oil. Note: This process can take 3 to 4 months.

Cocoa butter applied daily also helps, as does jojoba oil.

Soiled Soil

It is essential to take supplements of chromium, iodine and selenium since they are no longer in the food supply. These minerals were formerly in the soil and were absorbed by the plants, but the continual application of chemical fertilizers has removed these minerals from the soil. A chromium deficiency can make blood sugar problems worse. Iodine is needed for balanced thyroid activity, and selenium helps to regulate heart rhythm and protects against cancer.

Too Many White Blood Cells

Echinacea, a potent immune system stimulant, should not be administered to leukemia patients. Since echinacea works by causing white blood cells to multiply, and leukemia is a disease of the overproliferation of white blood cells, it is contraindicated in these cases.

Bioflavanoids For Cell Integrity

Bioflavanoids can be used to relieve swelling. They were formerly called vitamin P, which stood for permeability (allowing nutrients to permeate the cell wall). Bioflavanoids are also useful in the treatment of macula edema. Edema is retention of fluid in tissues and is caused by the cell wall's inability to regulate the passage of fluids in and out of the cell.

Essential Facts About Vitamin A

The body makes Vitamin A from beta-carotene. This type of Vitamin A is non-toxic to the system because the body will utilize only what it needs. If you consume too much Vitamin A from fish oil, it can be toxic. Anyone using this form should be closely supervised by their nutritionist. The maximum amount taken daily should be no more than 50,000 I.U.

Safe Licorice

Licorice root is good for detoxifying the liver and stimulating the adrenal glands. However, people tend to shy away from licorice because it raises blood pressure. The deglycyrrhizinated form of licorice does *not* raise blood pressure.

Cod Liver Oil Danger

People with liver disease should not take more than 25,000 I.U. of Vitamin A derived from fish liver oil, unless under a doctor's care, because it causes too much strain on the liver.

Kidney Problem Warning

Those with kidney problems should not take high amounts of potassium or magnesium, since these minerals overtax weakened kidneys.

Herpes Prevention

For prevention of cold sores or genital herpes, take 1000 to 2000 mg of lysine daily. During an outbreak, use 3000 to 6000 mg. Animal products contain lysine. Avoid arginine, another amino acid found in nuts, beans, chocolate and grains, because it can make the problem worse.

Kidney Transplant Aid

Kidney transplant patients who take immune suppressant drugs to prevent rejection get better results if they take fish oil supplements and zinc. Fish oil and zinc reduce the amount of cyclosporin these patients need to prevent rejection of their kidney transplants.

Seek A More Alkaline State

To insure optimum health, a proper acid/alkaline balance must be maintained. The normal range is 7. Readings below 7 are acid, above are alkaline. A simple litmus paper saliva test can diagnose these levels.

Most diseases are caused by an overly acid condition. To rectify this, the body must be made more alkaline. A high vitamin D intake, calcium supplementation, cod liver oil up to 7000 I.U., and foods such as eggs, fish, fortified milk, barley green, wheat green and sunflower seeds can accomplish this.

Safety Of Supplements

According to the Centers for Disease Control, no deaths have ever occurred from side effects of supplements.

Cayenne Red Pepper—New Miracle Drug

Heart attacks—Cayenne acts as a vasodilator in the coronary arteries allowing stronger blood flow.

Those who eat the most cayenne have the least incidence of heart disease and colon cancer.

Combined with garlic, cayenne relieves heart palpitations and fibrillation.

Cayenne raises the metabolic rate, producing heat which burns off more calories (thermogenics).

Applied to cuts, cayenne stops bleeding instantly.

Cayenne relieves constipation.

Mix cayenne powder with olive oil and apply it to the soles of the feet to relieve poor circulation or cold feet.

Cayenne works instantly as an energy stimulant.

Cayenne can be added to food or obtained in capsule form. If you experience a burning sensation, you can buffer it by mixing two parts cayenne to one part ginger.

Memory Drug

The most frequently recommended drug in Germany and France is ginkgo biloba, an herb that stimulates circulation in the brain, improving memory.

Autism

Autism can be due to a B-complex deficiency or a mineral imbalance.

Supplement Schedule

Vitamin E and iron supplements should not be taken at the same time, because they slow down each other's absorption.

Copper and zinc can displace one another.

Calcium and magnesium should be taken in the ratio of two parts magnesium to one part calcium.

Problematic Oil-Base Supplements

Some people get indigestion from supplements in an oil base. They should take the mycellized form (the dry form), but in order to get the same benefit as the oil-based supplement, they have to take twice as much of the dry form.

Herbal Facts

Aspirin is derived from white willow bark.

Hawthorne can be used to control blood pressure.

Ginger prevents vertigo and motion sickness.

Echinacea has anti-viral properties.

Guguloo is an Indian ayurvedic herb used to lower cholesterol.

Cinnamon shrinks fibroids.

Ephedra (Mormon tea) is a decongestant.

Helpful Herbs For The Heart

- Cayenne
- Hawthorne
- Kelp
- Motherwort
- Rosemary

- Turmeric (Curry contains turmeric)
- Valerian

Herbs To Enhance The Immune System
- Astragalus
- Echinacea
- Ginseng
- Pau D'Arco
- Yerba-Maté

Herbs For Diabetes
- Blueberry
- Goldenseal
- Gymnema-Sylvestra

Herbs For The Gastrointestinal System
- Dandelion Root
- Gentian
- Ginger Root
- Licorice Root
- Milk Thistle
- Schisandra
- Turmeric

Herbs For Heart Palpitations
- Hawthorne
- Valerian Root

Herbal Tea—Most Potent Form

Herbs in extracted form (liquid) are not the most effective because the extraction process leaves some of the product behind. It is best to take herbs in the form of tea.

Best Herbal Combination

One of the best herbal combinations for chronic fatigue is goldenseal, echinacea, astragalus and burdock root.

Ginseng Aids AIDS

AIDS and cancer patients lose the ability to produce gamma inteferon (an immune system stimulant). Ginseng aids in the production of inteferon.

Constipating Calcium

Calcium carbonate (from oyster shells) can cause constipation.

Counteract Prednisone

Patients who are prescribed large doses of prednisone for long periods of time should also take calcium with Vitamin D and magnesium to prevent bone loss caused by the prednisone.

Counteract Antibiotics

If you are on antibiotics, take acidophilus to maintain normal bacterial flora and prevent yeast infections.

Prevent Kidney Stones

To prevent kidney stones when taking high amounts of vitamin C, take B^6 and magnesium citrate, and drink plenty of water.

Zap Septicemia

Echinacea is effective for treating septicemia (blood poisoning).

Benefits Of Goldenseal

Apply goldenseal topically to large open wounds. It has antiseptic, antiviral and antibacterial properties.

Different Ginsengs

Not all ginseng is the same. Most people think the herb is an energizer, but, depending upon what type it is, the effects are vastly different.

Siberian ginseng, Korean ginseng and American ginseng each have different properties.

Siberian ginseng is an immune system stimulant and is for long-term use to build up the anabolic processes of the body.

Korean ginseng is for energy and resistance to fatigue and should be used on a short-term basis only.

American ginseng is a sedative and relaxant.

On The Pill? Check B^6 Levels

Women taking birth control pills need extra vitamin B^6 since the pills block proper absorption of this vitamin which is needed for:

- Sodium/potassium balance
- Production of hydrochloric acid needed for digestion

Deficiencies of B^6 cause:

- Arthritis
- Certain types of anemia
- Cracks around the mouth and eyes
- Fluid retention
- Hair loss
- Heart disorders
- Increase in urination
- Learning disabilities
- Neuritis
- Numbness and cramps in arms and legs
- Visual disturbances

On Antibiotics? Take Acidophilus

Antibiotics eradicate the good bacteria in the colon which produce acid to control the bad bacteria. When the balance is upset, the bad bacteria take over, causing an imbalance in the flora of the colon, leading to conditions such as diarrhea, tinnitus, fever, vaginal discharge, spaciness and lower abdominal distention. Acidophilus, which is lactobacillus, works by producing the acid that will destroy the bad bacteria.

White Willow Bark

White willow bark (an herb) can be used in place of aspirin. Although not quite as effective, it has no side effects. White willow bark is also an effective astringent for women with heavy menstrual bleeding or fibroid tumors. It temporarily tightens or contracts tissues, slowing the discharge of mucous and blood.

Comfrey Comforts

The herb comfrey is effective in healing ulcers, but high doses for long periods of time can adversely affect the liver.

Shark Cartilage Dosage

The dosage for shark cartilage varies for various conditions.

Patients with active cancer should take one gram daily for every two pounds of body weight.

Those with pancreatic cancer have had excellent results taking 75 grams daily.

The maintenance dose for recovered cancer patients is 10 grams daily.

Arthritis sufferers should take 10 grams daily.

10 grams daily can shrink uterine fibroids.

Note—Each capsule contains ¾ of a gram or 750 micrograms.

Extra Benefit Of Shark Cartilage

Shark cartilage contains 13 percent calcium, so anyone taking this supplement is also getting their daily dietary amounts of calcium.

Thwart Osteoporosis And Aging

Five mg daily of DHEA alleviates osteoporosis and aging.

Vitamin C Protector

The reason for taking bioflavanoids with Vitamin C is that bioflavanoids protect Vitamin C from oxidation.

The Iron Connection

Anyone suffering from hemachromatosis (too much iron in the blood) should have a liver biopsy performed to make sure the liver is not damaged. The treatment for this condition is to donate blood. Be sure your multiple vitamin does not contain iron. Since high Vitamin C consumption enhances iron metabolism, patients with this condition should reduce Vitamin C intake. Since iron causes free radical damage, increase the amounts of other antioxidants such as Vitamins A, B-complex E, zinc, bioflavanoids and selenium.

Natural Calcium Channel Blocker

Calcium channel blockers are used for control of high blood pressure. Magnesium acts as a natural calcium channel blocker without any dangerous side effect (see page 207).

Don't Get Rancid

Without antioxidants, body fat becomes rancid, stimulating the production of free radicals which cause dysfunction of the cells and lead to disease. To prevent this, take antioxidants such as Vitamin A, C, E and selenium.

Shark Liver Oil

Squalene (shark liver oil) applied topically is an effective remedy for most skin conditions.

RDA's Not Valid

RDA's for vitamins and minerals are too low to begin with. Due to poor absorption of nutrients, older individuals especially need higher doses of supplements to maintain optimum health.

Arrest Gallstones

Taurine, 1000 mg four times daily on an empty stomach, thins the bile, making it less viscous and eliminating the formation of gallstones.

Hiatal Hernia

Deglycyrrhizinated licorice lozenges are effective for treating symptoms of hiatus hernia.

Vitamin E

Vitamin E is non-toxic and may be taken in doses as high as 50,000 International Units (under a physicians care). Usual recommended doses range from 400 to 1200 I.U. daily. Diabetics should be aware that Vitamin E can reduce insulin requirements. Vitamin E also decreases the amount of digitalis needed to regulate heart rhythm.

Raynaud's Syndrome

Vitamin E is useful in treating Raynaud's Syndrome.

Side Effects Of Supplements

Megadoses of individual supplements taken over a long period of time may cause deficiencies in other supplements and may also have an effect on medications and their dosages.

All practitioners should be well aware of the following information when recommending such supplements to their patients.

Choline

High doses can cause a B^6 deficiency.

Copper

Megadoses deplete zinc levels.

An excess has an adverse affect on the immune system.

Folic Acid

High doses should not be taken by anyone with convulsive disorders or hormone-related cancers.

Iron

An excess lowers the function of the immune system and can exacerbate arthritis.

Magnesium

If the kidneys are diseased, do not take more than 300 mg daily.

Manganese

Too much causes loss of iron.

Niacin

Use cautiously with severe diabetes, glaucoma, peptic ulcers or impaired liver function.

PABA

Excessive amounts can have a negative effect on the liver, kidneys, thyroid and heart.

Vitamin A

A deficiency can lead to loss of Vitamin C.

An overabundance can deplete calcium.

Vitamin B^1

Too much affects the thyroid by stimulating thyroxine production. High levels of thyroxine cause hyperthyroidism.

Too much increases insulin production.

High doses can cause a B^6 deficiency.

Vitamin B^6

Depletes zinc.

Should not be taken with L-Dopa (medication used for Parkinson's Disease).

Vitamin C

Reverses the anticoagulant activity of the blood thinner Warfarin (Coumadin).

Megadoses can wash out B^{12} and folic acid.

Reduces the necessary dosage of medication for diabetes and heart disease.

Can change results of laboratory tests for sugar in the blood and urine.

Gives false negative results for blood in stools. (Horseradish and beefsteak also do this.)

Vitamin D

Raises calcium levels.

Depletes magnesium levels.

Milk that contains synthetic D depletes magnesium. All milk bought in supermarkets contains synthetic D.

High amounts can suppress the immune system.

An overabundance can create harmful calcium deposits in the blood vessels.

Vitamin E

Use cautiously with overactive thyroid, diabetes, high blood pressure or rheumatic heart disease (imbalance of the two sides of the heart).

Do not take with inorganic iron (ferrous sulfate).

Diabetics taking synthetic insulin can reduce the dosage by taking Vitamin E.

Raises sodium levels.

Zinc

Megadoses cause iron and copper loss.

If added to regime, be sure to get enough Vitamin A because these two supplements work better together.

Reduces sodium, E and potassium levels.

Calories In Fish Oil

Liquid supplements of fish oil and cod liver oil contain nine calories per teaspoon and 27 per tablespoon.

Wake Up Your Adrenals

The best supplements to support exhausted adrenal glands are licorice root and pantothene.

Ginseng Warning

Siberian ginseng is high in estrogens and may be dangerous for women with female cancer problems.

Protective Sleep Enhancer

The hormone, melatonin, in addition to being a sleep enhancer is also an oncostatic agent which protects against breast cancer. It is also a good source of serotonin.

Eat Prunes Instead

Mineral oil taken internally for its laxative effect stops the absorption of vitamins and minerals, preventing them from being metabolized by the system.

Flawed Finnish Study

In the spring of 1994, a study was published in *The New England Journal of Medicine* deriding the use of beta-carotene for protection against cancer in smokers.

In Finland, 27,000 smokers who smoked an average of one pack daily for 37 years were given 25,000 units of beta-carotene and 50 to 100 units of Vitamin E. After the six year study was completed, it showed 18 percent had more cancer than at the beginning of the study. The contention of the orthodoxy is that beta-carotene and other antioxidants are useless as a protector against cancer and may in fact even cause cancer.

Further investigation of the facts show the study was flawed and the conclusions taken out of context.

Fact 1. Beta-carotene should be taken in much higher amounts (100,000 I.U.) and 800 to 1200 I.U. of Vitamin E should have been used.

Fact 2. Vitamin C, which was not given, is the necessary vitamin to aid the liver in converting beta-carotene to Vitamin A.

Fact 3. Of all the European countries, Finland has the worst health and the highest rate of alcoholism. Therefore, many of the participating smokers were also heavy drinkers which causes a weakening of the liver's final conversion of beta-carotene to Vitamin A.

Fact 4. Since these smokers thought they were protected by the beta-carotene, many believed they could smoke even more. This caused further damage to their lungs.

Fact 5. Since the participants had been smoking for several years prior to the 6 year test, it is conceivable that many already had a precancerous condition.

Fact 6. There was no measurement of the blood levels of beta-carotene in these participants at the beginning of the study. Supplements of beta-carotene of 25,000 units daily will do nothing to protect an individual against cancer if the blood levels of beta-carotene are already high. Beta-carotene works synergistically with other antioxidants to protect against cancer. Alone, it is ineffective, and no other antioxidants were given to the participants, with the exception of Vitamin E in doses too small to be effective.

Fact 7. The beta-carotene used in the study was synthetic and it is well-known that synthetic beta-carotene does not have the protective properties of natural beta-carotene.

Fact 8. Since the study made the statement that beta-carotene can now cause cancer, the average American eating carrots, green peppers, green leafy vegetables, cabbage, and broccoli would then be subjected to cancer because these vegetables all contain large amounts of the so-called cancer-causing beta-carotene.

Fact 9. A carcinogenic dye, quinelene yellow, was added to the beta-carotene used in the study.

Fact 10. The Finnish soil is very low in selenium, and selenium must be given with beta-carotene for optimum protection.

Fact 11. Finland was one of the first European countries to receive heavy fallout from the Chernobyl disaster.

Fact 12. For full effectiveness of beta-carotene, the liver should convert it into Vitamin A, which is utilized as needed by the body, and any excess is eliminated. Vitamin A, derived from fish oil taken orally, can accumulate in the liver and cause toxicity. The beta-carotene levels in these patients were 1700 times higher than normal which shows it never converted into Vitamin A. If the beta-carotene had been given in a natural, rather than synthetic, form this would not have been the case.

200 other studies have shown that beta-carotene was effective in causing remission of cancer (one of the most successful and well-known of these studies was the China Study). This was never publicized in the media and there appears to be a flagrant misinterpretation of the facts.

Fact 13. If the skin color turns yellowish-orange, it implies the liver is not performing the proper conversion. Some of the participants' skin turned orange.

Fact 14. The systems of chronic smokers are toxic to begin with, and the participants in the study had a false sense of security thinking they were protected by the beta-carotene, which led them to overindulge in their addiction.

Fact 15. Vitamin C, an antioxidant, is needed to protect the body against free radicals and since smokers lose 25 mg of Vitamin C for every cigarette smoked, a two-pack-a-day smoker loses 1000 mg of Vitamin C daily. Interestingly enough, the RDA for Vitamin C is only 60 mg daily. Therefore, these participants had a severe Vitamin C deficiency which left them vulnerable to the overproliferation of cancer.

Conclusion. The fact that the Vitamin E, even in its small dosage, did protect these men against prostate cancer was *never* publicized.

As stated, hundreds of studies have shown the benefits of beta-carotene as a protector against cancer. Yet, one flawed study taken out of context and released by the pharmaceutical-backed media completely confuses the average lay person.

This has led to reduced sales of beta-carotene in the health food stores, which is exactly what the pharmaceutical companies desire, since beta-carotene is in the public domain and cannot be patented.

Flawed American Study

In January of 1996, newspapers all over the U.S.A. carried articles denigrating the use of beta-carotene. According to remarks made by Annette Dickenson, M.D., Director for Science and Regulatory Affairs of the Counsel for Responsible Nutrition, on Dr. Ronald Hoffman's January 20, 1996 radio program, the derogatory study, financed by the National Cancer Institute, was done on only one disease—lung cancer. In this study, *only* high risk people were used, including heavy smokers, cancer patients and those who had contact with asbestos. Dr. Dickenson also said that lung cancer can take 20 years to develop and this study was done over a four year period, which could have been after the cancer started to develop.

Beta-carotene given by itself is not as effective as when given in combination with other nutrients. Only one form of beta-carotene was given, and beta-carotene comes in multiple carotenoid forms. In addition, antioxidants work synergistically with each other. Beta-carotene protects other parts of the body from cancer, especially the prostate, and also helps prevent heart disease and cataracts.

Beta-carotene is converted into Vitamin A in the liver and those in the study could have had damaged livers from smoking or asbestos contact or existing cancers, preventing the beta-carotene from converting to Vitamin A in the liver, and thereby eliminating its positive effects.

Dr. Hoffman stated on his program that Richard D. Klausner, Director of the National Cancer Institute, "jumped the gun" and reported on the study before it was published. Hoffman said Chinese studies have shown *great* benefits using beta-carotene in other cancers, specifically esophageal and stomach cancer.

Charles Hennekens, Chief of Preventive Medicine at Brigham and Women's Hospital, stated that supplements are no substitute for a healthy diet.

However, there is no such thing as a healthy diet. Most foods in the market contain pesticides, herbicides and fungicides which cause depletion of nutrients. Canned foods contain preservatives which cause a deficiency of oxygen in the body's cells which can lead to disease. When frozen foods defrost, the cells rupture, causing rancidity of oils in the food.

Further, by the time food is purchased, it could be two weeks old. Tomatoes are picked green and matured by exposing them to certain heated gases. These gases are toxic to the body. Cooking food depletes it of most nutrients. Most people over age 45 have poor digestion which leads to poor absorption.

In addition, no mention was made in the study regarding the status of the participants in the placebo group.

Ring Out The New Ear

500 mg of niacin taken three times a day can relieve tinnitus (ringing in the ears). Niacin's side effect of flushing in the upper body, which may last for 20 minutes, is no cause for alarm.

Ginger Root

Ginger root is good for digestion and vertigo.

Mycellized Vitamins

Mycellized vitamins are much more powerful than regular supplements. Take one-half the amount you would of the unmycellized type.

Sulfite Neutralizer

Molybdenum, a mineral, is effective for reactions to the sulfites found in salads at some salad bars and in certain wines.

Poor Combination

Magnesium and calcium should be taken at different times of day since both compete for the same absorption sites on the cell. It is best to take the magnesium in the morning and the calcium in the evening.

Gentian

Gentian (an herbal remedy) is useful for treating yeast infections. It is also an excellent remedy for digestive problems.

Let The Sun Shine In

Studies have shown that Vitamin D helps prevent colon cancer. Twenty minutes of sun daily aids in the body's production of Vitamin D.

OJ Not Strong Enough

The average American consumes only 50 percent of the RDA for Vitamin A and 40 percent of the RDA for Vitamin C. These RDA's are already dangerously low. In order to receive the optimum amount of Vitamin C without supplementation, an individual would have to drink 300 glasses of orange juice daily.

RDA's

RDA's are designed for surviving, not for thriving.

Vitamin C Misinformation

Latest studies in the *Journal of Urology* show that a high amount of Vitamin C does not cause kidney stones.

B^1 Robber

Vitamin B^1, the morale vitamin, is depleted by consuming raw fish, black or green tea, coffee, chlorinated water, alcohol and sugar.

Alfafa Plant Parts

When using alfalfa as a therapeutic supplement, be sure it is made from the leaves, not the root. Never use the seeds because they contain a poisonous substance.

Shark Cartilage Absorption Aid

For better absorption, take acidophilus when using shark cartilage.

Don't Travel Without It

Grapefruit seed extract is useful for treating parasites. When traveling it is more effective than prophylactic antibiotic medication which can cause solar sensitivity.

Selenium Not Toxic

By mistake, 30,000 mcg. of selenium were in a multiple vitamin. No one died or even got sick, which proves selenium toxicity is overrated.

Synthetic Progesterone

All *synthetic* progesterone is made from soybeans, and *most* people are allergic to soybeans.

Goldenseal

Goldenseal lowers blood sugar.

When Vitamins Are Not Recommended

Stop taking Vitamin C, Vitamin E and fish oil one week before surgery as they thin blood.

A And E Competition

Vitamins A and E compete for absorption. It is best to take them at different times of the day.

CoQ-10

CoQ-10 is one of the best free radical scavengers to prevent cell oxidation. The average dosage is 100 mg daily.

Orange Urine

The B^2 in a multi-vitamin/mineral supplement often turns urine an orange color. This is no cause for alarm.

Ineffective Echinacea

Echinacea, an immune system stimulant, is ineffective for autoimmune diseases such as rheumatoid arthritis, multiple sclerosis, lupus and scleraderma. The reason is that the immune system is *overactive* in these conditions.

Stagger Your Echinacea

Do not take echinacea for longer than three consecutive weeks or it will lose its effectiveness. You need to stop taking it for one week before resuming treatment.

Exercise Protection

Strenuous exercise produces free radicals. The best way to scavenge these is to take glutathione, an amino acid. The general maintenance dose is 100 mg daily.

Anti-Proliferator Vitamin

Vitamin A is classed as an anti-proliferator vitamin. In cases where there is overproliferation of cells (autoimmune) that cause disease in the body, and where there is a high white blood count, as in chronic lymphocyte leukemia, the Vitamin A will reduce the production of the white blood cells.

Arginine

The amino acid, arginine, is a building block for nitrous oxide which prevents arteries from going into spasm.

Herbal Flush

Marijuana is a fat-soluble substance and remains in the system four to five weeks after cessation. Cocaine and alcohol remain in the body three to four days. An herbal flush consisting of goldenseal, cayenne, rhubarb, buckthorn, dandelion root and burdock aids in removing residual amounts.

Zinc's Destination

The prostate and pancreas utilize more zinc than other body organs.

High Iron Levels

High iron levels can cause joint pain, heart problems and constipation. If high levels are present, be sure your multi-vitamin does not contain iron. Another way to reduce iron levels is to be a blood donor.

45 Uses Of Herbs

Alfalfa—Richest Source Of Trace Minerals

Appetite stimulant
Blood purifier
Diabetes
Fatigue
Kidney cleanser
Ulcers

Aloe Vera—First Aid Plant

Burns
Digestion
Hemorrhoids
Scar tissue

Bee Pollen

Energy
Hay fever
Longevity

Black Cohash

Asthma
Bronchitis
Hormone balance
Menopause
Whooping cough

Black Walnut Hulls
- Parasites
- Ringworm

Blessed Thistle
- Blood circulation
- Blood purifier
- Gallbladder
- Lactation
- Strengthens heart

Boneset
- Fever

Borage
- Anti-inflammatory

Burdock
- Blood purifier
- Eczema
- Gout
- Skin diseases

Capsicum (Cayenne)
- Arthritis
- Blood pressure regulator
- Circulation
- Strokes
- Ulcers

Cascara Sagrada
- Constipation
- Gallbladder
- Intestines
- Liver disorders

Catnip
- Convulsions
- Diarrhea

Gas
Nerves

Celery
Acid neutralizer
Arthritis

Chamomile
Appetite stimulant
Insomnia
Nervousness

Chaparral
Blood purifier
Cancer
Tumors

Chickweed
Appetite depressant
Blood purifier
Helps dissolve plaque
Obesity
Ulcers

Comfrey
Boils
Fractures
Lungs
Swelling

Cornsilk
Bladder
Kidneys
Heart

Damiana
Increases sperm count
Menopause

Parkinson's Disease
Sexual stimulant
Strengthens ova

Dandelion
Blood purifier
Liver problems
Lowers blood pressure

Devil's Claw
Arthritis
Blood purifier
Diabetes
Gout

Dong Quai (Queen Of All Female Herbs)
Hot flashes
Internal bleeding
Menopause
Regulates menstruation

Echinacea (King Of The Blood Purifiers)
Antibiotic
Infections
Stimulates immune system

Ephedra
Bronchial dilator
Decongestant

Evening Primrose Oil And Borage Oil
Anti-inflammatory (hormone-like substances)
Controls arthritis
Dilates blood vessels
Lowers blood pressure
Prevents inflammation
Produces prostaglandins (hormone like substances)
Reduces cholesterol

Relieves pain of angina
Stops growth of numerous kinds of cancer cells
Stops thrombosis

Eyebright
Blood cleanser
Eye disorders
Liver stimulant

Fennel
Gas
Intestinal problems
Sedative for children

Fenugreek
Bronchial catarrh
Dissolves cholesterol
Dissolves mucous
Lung infections

Flaxseed
Constipation

Garlic (Nature's Antibiotic, Also Called Russian Penicillin)
Cancer
Heart disease
High blood pressure
Immunity
Intestinal worms
Parasites

Ginger
Circulation
Congestion
Fever
Headaches
Morning sickness of pregnancy

Nausea
Respiratory system
Seasickness

Ginseng (King Of The Herbs—The Cure-All Herb)
Antidote to various drugs and toxic chemicals
Enhances heart and circulation
Fatigue
Improves brain cells
Improves hearing and vision
Increases self-confidence
Lightens age spots
Lowers cholesterol
Normalizes blood pressure
Overcomes stress
Prevents arteriosclerosis
Protects body against radiation
Slows the aging process
Weakness

Goldenseal
Antibiotic
Liver problems
Infections

Gotu Kola
Depression
Food for the brain
High blood pressure
Mental fatigue
Senility

Hawthorne
Angina
Arrhythmias
Breathlessness
Congestive heart failure
Enlarged heart

Heart disease
Heart palpitations

Hops
Appetite stimulant
Delirium
Headache
Nervousness
Reduces excessive sexual desire

Horehound
Asthma
Coughs
Expectorant
Hoarseness
Laryngitis
Lungs

Horseradish
Appetite stimulant
Circulation
Sinus problems
Tumors
Worms

Horsetail
Coagulation
Circulation
Chilblains
Helps fractures heal
Nails

Hyssop
Lung ailments
Mucous expectorant
Poor digestion
Produces sweating

Irish Moss

Bronchitis
Contains iodine
High nutrient content
Prevents wrinkles
Softens skin

Jojoba

Chapped skin
Dandruff
Psoriasis
Scars

Juniper

Eliminates uric acid
Dropsy
High in natural insulin

Kelp

Complexion
Goiter
Obesity
Thyroid

Licorice

Addison's disease
Chest complaints
Contains estrogen
Drug-withdrawal symptoms
Laxative
Stimulates adrenal glands

Lobelia

Asthma
Bronchitis
Epilepsy
Expectorant
Food poisoning

Lungs
Miscarriage
Worms

Mandrake—Caution—Not To Be Used During Pregnancy

Aids female fertility
Chronic liver disease
Constipation
Fevers
Worms

Marshmallow

Asthma
Emphysema
Kidneys
Whooping cough

Mistletoe

Circulatory system
Heart stimulant
Migraines
Natural tranquilizer
Raises low blood pressure
Reduces cerebral activity
Spleen stimulant

Mullein

Earache
Insomnia
Loosens mucous
Narcotic properties without being addictive
Painkiller
Tuberculosis

Myrrh

Antiseptic
Bad breath
Colon

Hemorrhoids
Mouth sores
Sore throat
Stomach

Nettle

Arthritis
Diarrhea
High in chlorophyll
High blood pressure
Neutralizes uric acid

Papaya

Blood clotting agent
Digestion
Gas
Insect bites
Topical application of juice dissolves corns, warts and pimples

Parsley

Contains a substance in which cancer cells cannot multiply
Conjunctivitis
Could bring on labor pains
Helps dry up breast milk
Jaundice
Mild diuretic
Venereal disease

Passion Flower

Convulsions
Dimness of vision
Hyperactive children
Inflamed eyes
Insomnia
Menopause

Pennyroyal—Not To Be Used During Pregnancy

Applied externally acts as insect repellent
Flea control
Gas
Induces abortions (Caution—can cause serious problems)
Induces sweating
Leprosy
Menstrual enhancer

Peppermint

Appetite
Brings oxygen into the bloodstream
Convulsions
Digestion
Heartburn
Shock
Stomach sedative
Strengthens heart muscle

Psyllium

Diverticulitis
Intestinal cleanser
Intestinal lubricant

Red Clover

Blood purifier
Cancer
Nerve tonic
Rickets
Salve for burns
Sore eyes
Tremors

Red Raspberry

Enriches colostrum
Helps reduce false labor pains
Nausea
Strengthens uterine wall

Vomiting

Sage
Aids concentration
Excessive secretion of saliva
Gums
Mental exhaustion
Mouth infections
Mucous discharge

St. Johnswort
Depression
Internal bleeding
Leg ulcers
Loosens mucous
Painful menstruation
Wound healing

Sarsaparilla
Glandular balance
Increases metabolic rate
Progesterone production
Skin diseases
Testosterone production

Sassafras
Acne
Appetite control
Pain reliever
Psoriasis
Venereal disease

Saw Palmetto
Enlarged prostate
Reproductive organs
Sex stimulant
Suppresses weight increase

Skullcap

Convulsions
High blood pressure
Infertility
Insomnia
Nerves
Regulates sexual desire
Skin diseases

Senna

Increases intestinal peristalsis
Jaundice
Worms

Slippery Elm

Aids milk digestion
Assists activity of adrenal glands
Asthma
Diaper rash
Neutralizes stomach acid
Sore throat

Spearmint

Colic
Morning sickness

Taheebo (Pau D'Arco)

Antibiotic
Antiviral
Blood builder
Cancer
Relieves pain
Yeast infections

Thyme

Anemia
Body parasites
Fungal infections

Gout
Intestinal disturbances
Sciatica

Uva Ursi
Bright's disease
Diabetes
Gonorrhea
Increases urine flow
Tones urinary passages

Valerian
Convulsions
Hypochondria
Insomnia
Pain
Tranquilizer

White Oak Bark
Hemorrhoids
Internal bleeding
Mouth sores
Varicose veins
Worms

Wild Yam
Colic
Glandular balance
Prevents miscarriage

Willow Bark
Eczema
Functions like aspirin
Headaches
Sexual depressant

Yellow Dock
Blood purifier

Itching
Skin ailments

Yucca
Arthritis
Precursor of cortisone

Part IV

46 Understand Your Blood Tests

THE CHEM 24 TEST is done on the serum portion of blood and includes:

Glucose

Measures sugar levels.

Average range — 65 to 110.

Uric acid

Measures waste from protein metabolism.

Average range — 4.0 to 8.0.

Cholesterol

Measures liver and bile function, intestinal absorption, and assesses risk of arteriosclerosis.

Average range — 150 to 225.

Triglyceride Test

Measures blood fats sensitive to dietary intake, particularly that of refined sugar.

Average range — 40 to 175.

Calcium

Relates to bone metabolism, fat and protein absorption.

Average range — 9 to 10.8.

Phosphorous

Associated with calcium metabolism, bone and parathyroid function.

Average range — 2.5 to 4.5.

Total Protein Test

Building blocks of the body.

Average range — 6.0 to 6.8.

Albumin

Measures protein produced in the liver. Its primary function is maintaining pressure of blood vessels.

Average range — 3.2 to 5.0.

Globulin Test

Measures protein involved in antibody formation.

Average range — 1.5 to 3.5.

A/G Ratio Test

Indicates function of body's defense system.

Average range — 1.1 to 2.5.

Bilirubin Total Test

Measures breakdown products of red blood cells. Levels are increased in cases of liver disease.

Average range — 0.1 to 1.2.

Bilirubin Direct

A specific test for liver function. Elevated levels are usually caused if gallstones or tumors are present.

Average range — 0 to 0.5.

Bilirubin Indirect

Measures red blood cell breakdown and liver function.

Average range — 0.1 to 1.2.

BUN (Blood Urea Nitrogen)

Measures ability of kidney and liver to rid body of waste products from protein metabolism.

Average range — 10 to 25.

Creatinine Test

Measures muscle metabolism and kidney excretion.

Average range — 0.7 to 1.3.

BUN/Creatinine Test

An index of kidney function.

Average range — 10 to 35.

Sodium Test

Sodium is the electrolyte which offsets kidney activities for the discharge of toxins. It is essential for adrenal gland function and maintenance of the calcium to phosphorous ratio.

Average range — 135 to 147.

Potassium

Maintains heart rate, general muscle strength and normal nerve impulses.

Average range — 3.5 to 5.5.

Chloride Test

Shows adrenal, kidney, bladder and bowel function.

Average range 95 to 110.

CO_2 Test (Carbon Dioxide)

Measures cellular toxic waste.

Average range — 24 to 30.

LDH (Lactic Dehydrogenase)

A liver test that measures the enzyme associated with carbohydrate metabolism.

Average range — 60 to 225.

SGOT

A liver test that measures the enzyme associated with protein metabolism.

Average range — 0 to 55.

SGPT

A liver function test.

Average range — 0 to 45.

Alkaline Phosphatase

Measures metabolism of bone, liver and tumors.

Average range — 30 to 110.

ADDITIONAL BLOOD TESTS

Iron

Determines formation of red blood cells, hemoglobin and body growth.

Average range—50 to 150.

T4—Thyroxin

A measurement of the thyroid hormone essential for fat and protein digestion, absorption, growth and endocrine function.

Average range — 5.0 to 13.

SED (Sedimentation Rate)

A test for infectious processes in the body.

Average range — Men — 0 to 9. Women — 0 to 20.

HDL — High Density Lipoproteins (The Good Cholesterol)

Helps transport excess cholesterol to the liver for excretion.

Average range — 30 to 85.

LDL — Low Density Lipoproteins (Bad Cholesterol)

Measures fat and protein combination in the bloodstream that can adhere to the artery wall.

Average range — 60 to 180.

Complete Blood Count (CBC)

WBC — white blood cells; show the body's immune system function.

Average range — 4.8 to 10.8.

RBC — red blood cells; transport oxygen, glucose, carbohydrates, fats and proteins to the cells and remove carbon dioxide and normal metabolic poisonous wastes.

Average range:

Men — 4.6 to 6.2.

Women — 4.2 to 5.4.

Types And Percentages Of White Blood Cells

Segmented Neutrophiles

Measure the body's ability to fight infection.

Average range — 40 to 62 percent.

Lymphocytes

Fight Infection.

Average range — 30 to 38 percent.

Band Neutrophiles

Appear in impending infection.

Average range — 0 to 5 percent.

Monocytes

White blood cells that handle normal tissue breakdown.

Average range — 0 to 6 percent.

Eosinophiles

White blood cells vital for the preservation of life (immune system).

Average range — 0 to 5 percent.

Basophiles

Involved in intestinal allergies, skin eruptions, sinus, asthma and parasites.

Average range 0 to 2 percent.

TYPES AND PERCENTAGES OF RED BLOOD CELLS

HGB — Hemoglobin

Measurement of the oxygen and carbon dioxide carrying component of the red blood cells.

Average range:

Men — 14 to 18.

Women — 12 to 16.

HCT — Hematocrit

Measures the portion of percentage of blood that is made up of red blood cells.

Average range:

Men — 42 to 52 percent.

Women — 37 to 47 percent.

MCV — Mean Corpuscular Volume

Determines average size of blood cells.

Average range:

Men — 80 to 90.

Women — 79 to 97.

MCH—Mean Corpuscular Hemoglobin

Measures weight of red blood cells.

Average range 27 to 31.

MCHC — Mean Corpuscular Hemoglobin Concentration

Measures the percent of hemoglobin in each red blood cell.

Average range — 32 to 36 percent.

47 Acid/Alkaline Balance

Certain diseases are caused by an imbalance in the pH factor (acid/alkaline). Oriental medicine refers to Yin and Yang, Yin being acid and Yang alkaline. Anabolic means alkaline. Catabolic means acid. An imbalance between the two can be caused by the following factors:

Foods

Fruits, legumes and vegetables make the body more alkaline.

Meats, grains and nuts put the body in a more acid state.

Overconsumption of either of these foods types causes an imbalance. For instance, vegetarians' systems tend to be alkaline.

Nutrients

Sodium, potassium and chloride cause an alkaline state.

Calcium, magnesium, oxygen, sulfur and selenium cause an acid state.

Exercise

Aerobic exercise makes the body more acid.

Stretching and yoga make the body more alkaline.

Weightlifting makes the body more acid.

Sleep

While sleeping, the body is more alkaline.

When awake and alert, the body is more acid.

If the body becomes too acid at night, it could cause insomnia. During the day an alkaline state can lead to low energy and interfere with concentration.

Menstrual Cycle

During the first half (progesterone phase) of the menstrual cycle the body is acid. During the second half (estrogen phase) the body is alkaline. Acidifying supplements such as magnesium, B^6 and GLA can be used to treat PMS.

Japan puts GLA in all their dairy products, while we only put Vitamin D in ours.

Effects Of A Too-High Acid State

Diarrhea
High body temperature
High cholesterol
Insomnia
Low blood pressure
Migraines
Recessed eyes
Rheumatoid arthritis
Slow heart rate
Ulcers
Water retention

Effects Of A Too-High Alkaline State

Constipation
High fluid output
Low body temperature
Osteoarthritis
Protruding eyes
Rapid heart rate
Seizures
Sleepwalking
Viral diseases

Foods To Make The Body More Alkaline

Alfalfa
Algae
Almonds
Beans
Coconut

Dairy products
Eggs
Fruit
Green leafy vegetables
Honey
Millet
Molasses
Most herbal teas
Refined grains
Sea vegetables such as dulce and kelp
Soy sauce

Supplements To Make The Body More Alkaline

Bioflavanoids
Choline
Folic Acid
Gamma Oryzanol
Inosine
Inositol
Octocosanol
PABA
Pantothenic acid
Rutin
Spirulina
Vitamins C, B^1, B^2, B^3, B^{15}
Vitamin K

Minerals To Make The Body More Alkaline

Chromium
Iron
Molybdenum
Potassium
Sodium
Zinc

Amino Acids To Make The Body More Alkaline

Arginine
Carnitine

Glutamine
Histadine
Lysine
Ornithine
Phenylalanine
Tryptophan
Tyrosine

Other Substances That Make The Body More Alkaline

Aspirin
Cholesterol
Cigarettes
Estrogen
Insulin
Morphine
Non-steroidal anti-inflammatories
Phenobarbital
Prednisone
Recreational drugs

Activities That Make The Body More Alkaline

Meditation
Sleep
Yoga

Foods That Make The Body More Acid

Cinnamon
Cloves
Corn
Cranberries
Flesh-type protein
Garlic
Ginger
Hard cheeses
Horseradish
Mayonnaise
Nuts
Pomegranates

Seeds
Spearmint
Tomatoes
Unsaturated oils
Vinegar
Whole grains

Supplements That Make The Body More Acid
Calcium
Copper
Germanium
Magnesium
Manganese
Selenium
Silicon
Vanadium
Vitamins A, D, B^6, B^{12}, CoQ-10

Amino Acids That Make The Body More Acid
Aspartic
Cysteine
Glutamic
Methionine
Taurine

Other Substances That Make The Body More Acid
Adrenalin
Antibiotics
Antifungal medication
Digitalis
Fatty acids
Liver extract
Oxygen
Progesterone
Testosterone

Activities That Promote An Acid State
Intensive exercise

48 Mineral Ratios Pertaining To Thyroid And Adrenal Function

THYROID

Calcium To Potassium Ratio

Calcium in excess slows thyroid.

Potassium in excess speeds thyroid.

Slow metabolism = high calcium.

Low potassium = high calcium.

The higher the calcium to potassium ratio, the more sluggish the thyroid.

Zinc and magnesium raise potassium levels.

Copper lowers potassium.

ADRENAL

Sodium To Magnesium Ratio

High sodium = adrenal hyperactivity

Low sodium = adrenal insufficiency.

High sodium in relation to magnesium = speeded up adrenals.

Stress = high sodium and potassium.

An excessively high sodium to potassium ratio indicates the body is producing more inflammatory hormones than anti-inflammatory hormones.

49 Body Types (Weight Control)

G GONADAL

Description

Heavy thighs
Large buttocks
Small waist

Food Cravings

Creamy
Spicy

Balancing

Decrease gonadal function
Stimulate pituitary and thyroid

Diet

Herbal tea — Red clover (also eases menstruation)

High amounts of fruit, vegetables, whole grains, cabbage, cheese and yogurt

Low fat, low protein

A Adrenal

Description

Large breasts
Pot belly
Thick arms and legs

Food Cravings

Red meats
Salty foods

Balancing

Decrease adrenals
Stimulate pituitary and thyroid

Diet

Herbal tea — Parsley — clears adrenals
High protein
Low carbohydrate
No fat

T Thyroid

Description

Middle fat (apple shaped)

Food Cravings

Starches
Sweets

Balancing

Reverse thyroid

Diet

Herbal tea — Raspberry — cuts cravings
High protein
Low carbohydrate

P Pituitary

Description

Baby face
Childlike fat

Food Cravings

Dairy products

Balancing

Stimulate adrenals

Diet

Herbal tea — fenugreek
Meat
Vegetables

50 Liver Activities

- Breaks down hormones.
- Converts lactic acid to fuel.
- Converts thyroid hormone thyroxin.
- Disposes of ammonia.
- Extracts B vitamins from food.
- Glucose tolerance factor.
- Gluconeogenesis — conversion of proteins into sugars.
- Main glucose buffer.
- Makes bile salts.
- Makes carnitine from lysine.
- Poison detoxifier.
- Produces cholesterol for body functions.
- Protein metabolism.
- Stores various nutrients.

Part V

51 Airplanes

Jet Lag

Melatonin is helpful for jet lag. Take 3 mg before bed for seven days prior to the flight and for seven days after to help reset the biological clock.

Radiation Exposure

Any six hour plane flight gives the body the same amount of radiation as a chest X-ray. If, during a flight, a solar flare occurs (this happens 10 to 15 times a year), the amount of radiation could increase by 1000 times. Solar flares last 24 to 36 hours. Take antioxidants for seven days prior to and following the flight to protect the body.

Air Quality

The air quality of economy class on a plane is one-tenth that of other areas such as first class and the cockpit. In order to save money, the air is recirculated. This is the reason so many people get sick after a flight. One person with an upper respiratory infection can contaminate the entire area.

Dangerous Low Humidity

During a long flight, the humidity can be as low as 0 percent. The average humidity in the Sahara desert is 20 percent.

Preventive Measures

Drink lots of water because water contains high amounts of oxygen.

Increase Vitamin C to at least 1000 mg three times a day.

Eat fruits and vegetables.

Limit caffeine and alcohol, which are further dehydrating.

52 Pets

Benefits Of Pets

Older people who have pets live longer and have lower blood pressure.

Pet Food

To enhance the health of your pet, use only food from the health food store since it is organic and devoid of by-products.

Supplements

Give all animals a multi-vitamin/mineral. It helps add years to their life and life to their years.

Dander Control

Individuals who are allergic to cats should bathe the cat to get rid of dander, the usual cause of their allergy. This statement also appears in the chapter on allergies, but since pets are so essential for many people's health and well-being, it is repeated here.

Mange

Add flaxseed oil to dog food to control mange and falling hair.

53 Testing Procedures

Danger Of Dental X-rays

Dental X-rays can cause cataracts through the manifestation of free radicals from the radiation. Patients are only covered from the neck down with a lead shield. For protection from the effects of radiation, take glutathione, bioflavanoids, Vitamin C, N.A.C. and selenium.

White Coat Syndrome

White coat syndrome (nervousness from being in a doctor's presence) has been known to elevate blood pressure readings. It can also elevate blood sugar and cholesterol readings.

Inadequate Testing

Conventional blood tests do not always give enough information to allow the physician to diagnose certain ailments properly. A 35-year-old woman was examined by an orthodox physician for symptoms relating to low blood sugar, overactive thyroid and Candida (yeast infection). Routine blood tests showed no abnormalities. The patient continuously complained of not feeling well, and was sent to a psychiatrist for evaluation. No serious psychological problems were found. After more futile follow-up visits to the physician, a friend of hers recommended she see me.

I took her history and discovered she was indeed suffering from overactive thyroid, candida and hypoglycemia (low blood sugar). Blood tests I recommended included thyroid auto antibody test, blood antibodies for immunoglobulins A, G and M and a 6 hour glucose tolerance test with insulin levels. These tests confirmed my analysis.

She followed the program I suggested and recovered. This case shows that many diagnostic procedures ordered by the orthodoxy are inadequate. Health care costs skyrocket when the patient is shunted from specialist to specialist.

Unnecessary Testing

Patients are often subjected to painful invasive diagnostic procedures in order to protect doctors against malpractice suits. These suits are initiated by lawyers interested only in their own financial rewards and not in the patients well-being.

Unnecessary X-rays

Most preoperative chest X-rays have been found to be unnecessary.

Side Effect Of Fasting

Bilirubin levels (an indicator of liver and spleen function in the breakdown of red blood cells) can rise when fasting (Gilbert's Syndrome).

Dangerous Contrast Medium

Barium, used in studies of the upper and lower GI tract, can cause obstructions if not completely eliminated.

Ultrasound Not Without Danger

Ultrasound, commonly used for prenatal studies, can have an effect on rapidly growing tissue such as a fetus.

Blacks "Benefit" By Racism

Because of racism, blacks in VA hospitals who did not receive as many sophisticated tests and procedures as whites, actually did better in the long run.

54 EDTA Chelation

The Many Facets Of Chelation

Chelation was first used to decrease lead levels in the body, and patients who underwent the procedure reported their angina pain had disappeared or decreased. EDTA chelation therapy is best known for its ability to remove plaque from the arteries. It is also beneficial for those with macular degeneration, intermittent claudication (leg cramps), gangrene, Raynaud's Syndrome (cold hands) and other micro-circulatory problems.

Natural Chelators

Natural oral chelators are Vitamin C, the sulfur-containing amino acids cysteine, methionine and alginate (kelp). These substances can be used in a maintenance program for good health but they don't take the place of EDTA chelation.

Get The Lead Out

If levels of lead in the blood are above five to ten parts per million, the lead should be chelated out of the body immediately.

Additional Benefits Of Chelation Therapy

Reverses macular degeneration.

Eliminates free radicals that cause aging.

Reverses osteoporosis by taking calcium out of the plaque and transporting it back into the bone.

55 Statistics

U.S. Compared To Other Industrialized Nations

Of the leading 19 industrial nations, the United States is # 1 in:

- Caesarian section births.
- Coronary bypass operations per capita.
- Deaths of children under age 5.
- Incidence of cancer among men.
- Medical malpractice suits.
- Percentage of infants born with low birth weight.
- Percentage of population without health insurance.
- Snack food consumption.
- Total health care spending.

The United States is tied for first place with four other countries for infant mortality, tied with two others for first place in calcium consumption accompanied by high rates of osteoporosis, and tied with four countries for first place in fat consumption.

The United States is 13th in public health spending and 15th in life expectancy.

Longevity Factors For Cancer Patients

Women with the same type of cancer as men live longer. Married men with the same type of cancer as single men live longer.

What Is The Killer?

Causes of the 2,148,000 deaths in the United States yearly are:

Table 1: Killer Diseases

Killer Disease	Number of Deaths
Heart Disease	720,000
Cancer	505,000
Strokes	144,000
Accidents	92,000
Lung Disease	87,000
Pneumonia and Flu	80,000
Diabetes	50,000
Suicide	31,000
Liver Disease and Cirrhosis	26,000
AIDS (top killer of young men between 25 and 40)	25,000

Table 2: Principal Causes Of Killer Diseases

Killer Cause	Number of Deaths
Tobacco	19% of all deaths per year, or 400,000
Diet activity patterns, including obesity	300,000
Alcohol	100,000

Safer On The Battlefield

During the Vietnam War, 50,000 lives were lost in nine years. But, each *year*, 300,000 Americans are killed in hospitals as a result of medical negligence, the most frequent causes being: Administering the wrong prescription or having the decimal point in the wrong place which gives the wrong dosage. This information comes from a 1,500 page report, put out by Ralph Nader's consumer advocate group, of a three year study which included the causes of death in American hospitals.

Brain Surgery Success Rate

Eighty percent of those operated on for malignant brain tumors die within a year.

Doctor Nature

Eighty-five percent of all minor illnesses are self-limiting. Therefore, rushing to a doctor without waiting for nature to take its course is an exercise in futility.

Recovery Doubtful

It is rare for older people to recover from diseases such as arthritis, cancer, multiple sclerosis, diabetes, lupus, Alzheimer's disease and hypertension. Taking into consideration all the medications administered and procedures performed, the overall success rate is extremely low.

Disregard For Public's Health

Of the 80,000 chemicals produced yearly in the United States, only 2 percent have been tested for their toxicity. 98 percent are discharged into the environment without a thorough evaluation of their safety. This is erring on the side of profit instead of health.

Lowering Testing Costs

Costs of diagnostic procedures for determination of clogged arteries are:

- Echocardiogram $800.00
- Thallium stress test (nuclear imaging) $1200.00
- Angiogram $4000.00
  (without complications or hospital stay)
- MRI $1200.00

One million angiograms are performed annually in the U.S. If MRI studies were done instead, $4 billion could be saved.

Popular Medication Fails

Latest studies have shown the overall death rate from heart disease has increased despite the wide use of cholesterol-lowering medication.

Pricey Health Care Fails

The United States spends one trillion dollars on health care yearly. This is twice the per capita amount of any other civilized country on earth. Despite this huge expenditure, Americans have among the world's highest incidences of heart disease, cancer, diabetes, osteoporosis, arthritis, neonatal disease and mental illness.

Put Your Values In The Right Place

The government spent $28 million to find out if swine (pigs) suffer emotionally before they are slaughtered. The total budget for alternative medical exploration is only $2 million.

Drug Side Effects In Elderly

- 61,000 elderly people suffer from drug-induced Parkinson's disease symptoms.
- 32,000 elderly people suffer hip fractures from drug-induced falls.
- 163,000 elderly people suffer from drug-induced memory loss.
- 659,000 elderly people are hospitalized due to adverse reactions to drugs.
- 31,000 elderly people are hospitalized for treatment of ulcers caused by arthritis medicatio.

In addition, there are hundreds of thousands of cases of drug-induced fainting spells.

Overmedicated Population

The number of legal prescriptions in the United States is 2.2 billion yearly. This overmedication is one of the causes for a secondary immune deficiency.

The Top 10 Items Sold In The United States

Marlborough Cigarettes

Coca Cola Classic
Pepsi
Kraft Processed Cheese
Diet Coke
Campbell Soup
Beer
Tide Detergent
Folgers Coffee
Winston Cigarettes

Prices For Medications

Table 3: Prices For Medications

Medication	Amount	Strength	Cost
Prozac	60	20 mg	$83.95
Zolot	60	50 mg	$116.95
Mevacor	60	20 mg	$109.14
Capiten	60	50 mg	$70.95
Diabeta	100	5 mg	$54.95
Diabenese	100	250 mg	$72.95

Note: The generic form of Diabenese, for example, costs $12.95 for the same amount.

Atmosphere Losing Oxygen

The ancient atmosphere contained 38 percent oxygen. In the United States today, it is down to 15 to 20 percent. The body has had to adapt to an atmosphere containing half the amount of oxygen necessary for optimum health. This has compromised the immune system and led to disease.

Intellect And Illness

A comparison of disease rates between high school dropouts and those who complete high school and have some college education shows the following:

Dropouts

- Five-fold increase in arthritis.
- Four and a half times the rate of high blood pressure.
- Three and a half times the rate of stomach ulcers.
- Four times the rate of diabetes.
- Four times the rate of kidney disease.
- Six times the rate of chronic bronchitis.
- Nine times the amount of heart attacks.
- Three times the rate of cancer.
- Twice the amount of tuberculosis.

Higher-Educated

More allergies.
Higher incidence of multiple sclerosis.

Doctor Heal Thyself

A nationwide study of the health habits of our country's medical doctors revealed:

- 55 percent are overweight by more than 10 pounds.
- 34 percent have blood cholesterol levels over 200.
- 22 percent chose beef for dinner over fish or chicken.
- 12 percent ate fish more than other animal protein.
- A male doctor's lifespan is only 58 years versus 73 years for the average American man.

Drug Price Increases

During a recent 5 year period, the inflation rate was 25 percent. However, the price of the nine top-selling drugs in the United States increased by the following percentages:

Zantac (ulcer medication)	38%
Prozac (anti-depressant)	58%
Premarin (Estrogen) #1 selling drug	85%
Mevacor (cholesterol-lowering medication)	27%
Ceclor (antibiotic)	56%
Zanax (tranquilizer)	78%
Seldane (antihistamine)	63%
Augmentin (antibiotic)	64%
Zoverax (antiviral)	47%

56 Better Late Than Never

Most of the following drugs have been *removed* from the market due to their harmful side effects and are no longer available. One can only wonder how many of todays "safe prescriptions" will be added to the list in the future.

Bendectin
Use - Nausea of pregnancy
Effect - Malformed babies

Reserpine
Use - Blood pressure
Effect - Carcinogen

Methotrexate
Use - Psoriasis
Effect - Anemia and Carcinogen

Urethene
Use - Leukemia
Effect - Carcinogen in liver, lungs and bone marrow

Milotane
Use - Leukemia
Effect - Necrosis of renal glands

Plaxin
Use - Tranquilizer
Effect - Deaths

Pronap
Use - Tranquilizer
Effect - Deaths

Clofibrate
Use - Lower cholesterol
Effect - Possible carcinogen

Stilboesterol
Use - Pregnancy
Effect - Loss of consciousness

Flamanil
Use - Cardiac tonic
Effect - Heart damage and deaths

Thalidomide
Use - Nausea of pregnancy
Effect - 3500 deaths and severly malformed babies

MER- 29
Use - cholesterol-lowering
Effect - Birth defects

Amydopyrine
Use - Painkiller
Effect - Lethal blood damage

Bismuth
Use - Diarrhea
Effect - Cerebral trouble and death

Part VI

57 Case Histories

The Future Has No Time For You

The average time a doctor spends with a patient in America is less than six minutes, so you should take control of your own health now!

The new rules that Washington will soon impose on us, this hotly debated health system, will be more cruel to human life. It will firmly place the individual second to the system and create a hostile new environment.

It will encourage, as *The New York Times* has reported, a medical "industry that uses equipment and procedures to cut costs and raise profits, often at the expense of the patient's health, that operates with few rules to assure quality care and that has induced doctors to play along by giving them a share of the cash."

The following case histories are only a RED ALERT for worse times to come.

Fear Takes Over

Women with first-degree relatives (mother and/or sister) who have had ovarian cancer are being advised to have their ovaries removed prophylactically. The medical system continues to bamboozle American women, frightening them into having procedures leading to problems that would not have occurred otherwise.

Sheila M. lost both her mother and sister to ovarian cancer and was living in fear for her life. She expressed this fear to her gynecologist who checked her every six months and always found her to be in perfect health. However, he recommended she have her ovaries removed, citing her family history and emotional state.

Although she was only 29, Shelia opted for the surgery. She was a single woman with a good career and was not interested in marriage or motherhood. Future side effects were not considered as no long-term studies had been performed on prophylactic complete hysterectomies.

She was told she would have to take estrogen for the rest of her life to protect her from heart disease and osteoporosis. Since her uterus was also removed, it was not deemed necessary to administer Provera (progesterone) which is used to prevent uterine cancer. Note: Provera should be prescribed even though the uterus is removed because the activity of estrogen in the body, if not buffered by progesterone, can cause cancer in the breasts.

The surgery was performed and her recovery was uneventful. The estrogen prescribed immediately caused weight gain and fluid retention. In order to alleviate the side effects, diuretic medication was prescribed which led to nausea and constant urination. More medication was prescribed to deter urination and alleviate nausea.

Shelia was unhappy about her physical condition and feeling remorse over having had the procedure. Four years down this medication-requiring-medication road, she developed severe abdominal pains. Post-operative scar tissue in her colon and bladder was blamed and further surgery was needed to correct this.

At the same time, they discovered multiple breast masses that were found to be estrogen receptive. Estrogen replacement therapy was stopped, and Tamoxifen, an antihormonal drug, was prescribed, which also stopped estrogen production in her liver, body fat, hair follicles, pineal gland and adrenals. She eventually developed liver toxicity leading to chronic fatigue and depression. Shelia was then referred to a psychiatrist who prescribed Prozac and Lithium.

This unnecessary nightmare attack on Shelia's body, mind and spirit was completely unnecessary and could have been avoided. Natural healing doctors have *great* success treating women at risk for ovarian cancer with a diligent nutritional program, a vitamin regimen, exercise and meditation. And they keep women out of hospitals.

Unnecessary Hysterectomy

Patricia H., a 42-year-old woman, became alarmed when she noticed staining in the middle of her menstrual cycle and sought medical attention. She made an appointment with her primary care physician who examined her and referred her to a gynecologist, who subsequently referred her to an oncology gynecologist.

After going through a battery of invasive tests, Patricia was diagnosed with severe endometriosis (functioning uterine tissue growing in parts of the body other than the uterus). She was relieved to learn that no malignancy was present, but alarmed by what the doctors told her would happen if she did not undergo a complete hysterectomy, including the removal of the uterus, cervix, ovaries and fallopian tubes.

She was told that, without the surgery, the endometriosis could eventually lead to a strangulation of her colon, bladder and kidneys and possible death. The terror this woman felt can never be fathomed by a person who has not been in a similar situation. The doctors insisted on performing the surgery within a week and stated that, if she waited, she would be dead within three months. Under these terrifying circumstances, she agreed to the procedure.

The average American woman is under the impression that the only way severe gynecological disorders can be treated is by removing her reproductive organs. This is not so. It is simply a matter of economics. A doctor is no different from any other kind of businessman. His object is to be successful no matter what the consequences.

The white-coated legions may, in some respects, be altruistic but far too many order extensive treatment without even considering a simpler procedure. The average patient goes into a state of shock over her diagnosis and can be easily coerced into having an operation that is a form of castration and destroys an integral part of her femininity.

A side effect of this surgery is the formation of scar tissue and lesions leading to obstructions in the small and large intestine, bladder and rectum. This information is never revealed to the patient, who later in life, could suffer severe complications that often require further surgery.

Terrified and believing she had no choice, Patricia opted for the surgery. Her recovery period was extremely painful physically and mentally, and the stress interfered in her relationship with her husband.

This is just one case among the thousands of unnecessary surgical procedures that fill the coffers of unscrupulous businessmen who once took an oath, "First do no harm." All of Patricia's physical and mental trauma could have been avoided if she had sought natural healing methods and learned how to flush out illness the natural way.

When women with endometriosis seek my advice, I investigate the *cause* of their problems instead of just treating the symptoms. and, most of the time, the cause is unopposed estrogen (overactive estrogen combined with low progesterone). Balancing their hormones usually alleviates the condition and saves the patients from surgery and the hospital.

Calculated Fear

A 60-year-old executive in excellent health who worked out regularly was convinced to undergo a complete physical by his tennis partner. A routine chest X-ray showed a suspicious area in the lower lung. Surgery was performed, and a benign lesion was removed.

The time period between the original X-ray and the surgery was two and a half months. Although the MRI and CAT scans had been negative, the doctors had been pessimistic. During this time, he developed abdominal distress due to anxiety and apprehension about the final diagnosis.

When the doctors said further testing for the abdominal complaints, including upper and lower GI X-rays, endoscopy and colonoscopy were necessary, he decided to take control of his illness and seek non-orthodox treatment with me.

I explained that the abdominal distress was due to his anxiety. Even though the lung biopsy had been negative, the unnecessary fear instilled in him had caused the abdominal pain and further testing would only have exacerbated the situation. Once he was able to relax, without having to endure further assaults on his body, his pain disappeared and he was able to return to his previously active lifestyle and avoid further hospitalization.

In its insistence on overdiagnosing diseases, the orthodoxy often causes other ailments in the body to proliferate.

Children Also Have Rights

Steven, a bright seven-year-old elementary school student, was so hyperactive that his learning ability was impaired and he was having problems relating to the other children. He couldn't sit still in class, had poor concentration, and his disruptive behavior prevented the teacher from fulfilling her obligations to the other children.

Steven's mother took him to the pediatrician who recommended a drug used to calm hyperactive children. The mother's personal experience with mood-altering medication had been very traumatic. She had become so depressed on it that she had to be institutionalized.

Not wishing to subject her son to the same traumatic experience, she inquired about other treatments. The options were medication, psychotherapy, or a combination of both. She decided to investigate further on her own and did some research at the public library where she discovered a book and video called *Is This Your Child?* by Dr. Doris Rapp.

The video described how an extract of a particular food the child was sensitive to could cause a Dr. Jekyll and Mr. Hyde personality change. The degree of change was very severe, and the child became so physically violent that he had to be restrained. The book and video further described how a simple change in the child's diet could eliminate the problem.

Most of the offending foods, in order of severity, were:

- Processed sugar products
- Milk
- Soy
- Citrus
- Grains

- Eggs
- Corn Syrup
- Other offenders were chemicals, preservatives and coloring agents.

The mother decided to try an elimination diet to find out what the offending foods were. Removing milk and sugar from Steven's diet changed his behavior pattern and his scholastic accomplishment so much that the teacher remarked to his mother about how well the medication was working.

Intelligence is no match for the propaganda heaped on the public by the pharmaceutical industry. Far too many highly educated people are brainwashed by the medical establishment.

The drugging of elementary school children acts as a precursor to the formation of hard drug addiction at a future date. Latest studies show drug addiction in teenagers and adults often starts with giving the child a "harmless" simple medication without considering its long-term side effects.

It is interesting to note this same medication is prescribed to depressed adults to cause the opposite effect (mood elevation and increased activity).

Beware Of Standard Procedures

Mrs. J. was astonished when her ophthalmologist informed her that cataracts would be removed from both her eyes at the same time. Her astonishment was not due to the fact that cataract surgery is usually performed on one eye at a time in order for the patient to maintain vision while the other eye heals. Mrs. J. is blind in one eye and could not fathom why a cataract should be removed from a sightless eye. When she questioned the doctor, she was told, "This is standard procedure."

In their zeal to do surgery, this is an everyday occurrence among unscrupulous practitioners. Pain, suffering and anxiety are all too often disregarded, and the monetary reward takes precedence.

When the doctor said it was standard procedure, Mrs. J. felt she was not being treated as an individual and decided to seek a second opinion from a holistic ophthalmologist. This doctor informed her that removing a cataract from her sightless eye would have no benefit and could possibly cause infection and disfigurement.

The cataract in her "good" eye did not require immediate removal, he told her, and could possibly be eliminated by stringent dietary practices along with supplementation. The most important factor was to decrease sugar consumption since glucose diffuses into the lens, forcing its metabolism to shift to the sorbitol pathway. This forms large amounts of sugar alcohol, increasing the influx of fluid into the lens which stretches the fiber, causing metabolic damage.

Her vitamin therapy consisted of high amounts of specific antioxidants and bioflavanoids. Mrs. J. was very anxious to avoid surgery, yet preserve the sight in her functioning eye, and adhered to the program. To her amazement, within weeks her vision began to increase and no hospitalization or surgery was necessary.

For further information about treating eye problems holistically, read *Nutrition And The Eyes* by William Sardi. 1-800-809-2219.

Harmful Medications

Interferon was prescribed to Joseph C. for treatment of hepatitis B (the most virulent form of hepatitis). The effectiveness of interferon for treating hepatitis is only 20 percent and unfortunately, in his case, it was not successful.

The hepatitis progressed, and when the doctors said there was no hope, he became severely depressed and was referred to a psychiatrist. After reviewing his case, the psychiatrist prescribed two anti-depressant medications. Joseph experienced severe side effects from these medications, including rapid heartbeat, hyperactivity, headaches and stomach pains.

The original problems with his liver continued and only palliative therapy was administered. He was unable to work and lost his job. This resulted in domestic stress, leading to more anxiety and depression along with further diminished health.

One of Joseph's daughters was a massage therapist who worked for a natural healing doctor with extensive experience treating patients with terminal illnesses, such as hepatitis, AIDS and cancer. She convinced her father that mainstream medicine was not helping him.

The alternative healing doctor examined Joseph and determined that his condition could be reversed by rebuilding the damaged liver cells. A detoxification program was immediately instituted. Following detoxification, selected nutrients were recommended to rebuild the damaged liver cells and aid in their return to normal function.

Within three weeks, the constant pain in his right upper abdomen decreased, his mood improved and he appeared to be well on the road to recovery. Two months later he showed so much improvement that he was able to return to work and his relationship with his family greatly improved.

This is another classic example of mainstream medicine prescribing ineffective, often harmful, medication that could endanger a patient's life. It is my fervent hope that, in the near future, mainstream medicine will overcome their prejudice against alternative healing therapy and be more accepting of natural modalities which can reduce surgery and hospital stays.

Duped By The Doctor

As part of her annual checkup, a 70-year-old woman was advised to have the blood levels of her cholesterol checked. She asked the doctor why, as she was in excellent health and had no apparent symptoms. The doctor insisted it was a routine procedure he recommended to all his patients.

The test he took showed her total cholesterol reading was high (275) with a low HDL (32). HDL is known as the good cholesterol. The doctor suggested she go on a low fat, high complex carbohydrate diet without being too specific about the details. The woman followed his advice as best as she could with the information given her.

Two months later she returned for a follow-up blood test which showed her cholesterol had increased to 295. She was quite baffled since she had been very careful about what she ate. The doctor recommended she take cholesterol-lowering medication.

She was disturbed about being prescribed a medication with so many known side effects and was reluctant to use it. However, the doctor insisted that, in order to maintain her health, it was necessary to lower her cholesterol medically, since the diet had not been effective.

Three weeks after she started the medication, her energy was so depleted she was unable to enjoy her daily activities. When she returned to the doctor, new blood tests showed her Vitamin B^{12} levels had dropped significantly. He explained that the low B^{12} levels were the cause of her fatigue and recommended B^{12} injections weekly. Despite the medication, her cholesterol had only dropped 12 points.

She could not understand the rationale of taking medication that left her too tired to take her daily walk when exercise is recommended to lower cholesterol levels. Yet the doctor insisted that, in order to prevent arterial damage from cholesterol build-up, it was critical for her to remain on the medication.

Out of desperation, the woman sought a different approach to control the situation without side effects. She had heard about alternative therapy practitioners having success with non-toxic treatments, but she had no idea where to find one. She inquired at a health food store, but due to FDA regulations, they were not allowed to offer a recommendation. The clerk suggested she look in the yellow pages under nutritionists.

She located a nutritionist who recommended a high protein, low carbohydrate diet. The nutritionist gave her a detailed explanation of the diet along with selected cholesterol-lowering supplements including niacin, fish oil, chromium picolinate, pantothene and lecithin, and a printed handout with information showing the difference between fats, carbohydrates and protein.

Contrary to the popular belief that fats and proteins raise cholesterol, the doctor informed her that high cholesterol was caused more often by carbohydrates (sugars) than by fats and proteins. By decreasing the amount of carbohydrates ingested, a person's cholesterol will burn as energy in place of sugars that were not consumed.

She stopped the medication, followed the dietary advice of the nutritionist and, much to her delight, within two weeks her energy increased and she was able to resume her previous physical activity and active lifestyle. Four weeks later, a blood test showed a 75 point drop in her total cholesterol and an increase of 15 points in her HDL. She continued to improve.

Fortunately this woman had only one side effect. Many people who are prescribed cholesterol-lowering medication suffer a combination of other debilitating side effects, particularly low absorption of vitamins A, D, E and K, leading to a multitude of deficiencies in the body that could eventually end in death.

Cholesterol-lowering medication stops all cholesterol absorption originally derived from food. Cholesterol is a sterol responsible for the production of many hormones such as progesterone, estrogen, adrenalin and insulin. Deficiencies in these essential hormones are extremely deleterious to health. Cholesterol is involved in the production of the material that covers all cells, allowing the transportation of essential material in and out of the cell.

Aside from the side effects that damage an individual's health and well-being, it is my opinion that these medications increase business for doctors by causing other ailments that require patients to spend time and money unnecessarily.

Pawns Of The Pharmaceutical Companies

Pamela S, a 24-year-old water meter reader, developed a severe cold that lingered. She purchased an over-the-counter cold remedy that contained a combination of an antihistamine and a decongestant. The cold symptoms abated somewhat, but she experienced side effects of severe lethargy, fatigue, dry eyes and mouth. She had to drink so much water that she was forced to spend an inordinate amount of time seeking rest rooms and was unable to accomplish her normal work schedule.

Her nose stopped running, but when she developed severe sinus pressure, Pamela decided to seek medical attention. Her primary care doctor prescribed an antibiotic which was ineffective and caused a yeast infection, a known side effect. She still had the cold and also developed a vaginal discharge and severe itching, along with bloating in her lower abdomen and a white coating on her tongue. She was becoming so forgetful that she couldn't remember the numbers on the meter long enough to write them down.

She tried an over-the-counter remedy for the itching in her vaginal area. It alleviated the condition for a week, but it recurred after her menstrual period. She returned to the primary care physician who then referred her to a gynecologist, who prescribed systemic anti-yeast medication. A few weeks after taking the medicine, she developed a pain in her upper right abdominal area accompanied by high fever and severe diarrhea.

The gynecologist then ordered blood tests which showed abnormally high liver enzymes. Pamela was admitted to the hospital where further tests showed lesions had formed on her liver, causing hepatitis, a serious malady which can lead to death.

In an attempt to find a solution to the problem, a conscientious physician who believed in natural healing methods questioned her closely about the medications she had been using. He was astounded to learn she was still taking the anti-yeast medication. He immediately cancelled her prescription and prescribed instead high amounts of the natural product, lactobacillus acidophilus, which balanced the bacterial flora in her intestines and colon and got rid of the poisonous residue from the yeast infection. This allowed the liver to repair itself and resume its detoxifying action in the body.

Pamela is fortunate that a doctor who refused to be a pawn of the pharmaceutical companies was assigned to her case because the acidophilus he gave her was effective in controlling the yeast infection. If she had not taken the antihistamines for the cold in the first place, her own nasal secretions would have flushed out her sinuses rather than drying out her tissues and leaving them open for an infection to take hold.

This is an all-too-frequent example of a medication that is supposedly not harmful leading to a series of events that were not necessary, that harmed the patient and added to the high cost of health care.

Every knowledgeable nutritionist knows that, when taking antibiotics, it is essential to take acidophilus. Most of the orthodoxy pays no attention to this and, in a sense, actually causes other illnesses without taking the patient's best interest to heart.

Oh Well, Just Another Misdiagnosis

Jennifer, a 63-year-old food service employee, contracted a severe debilitating virus. She was so incapacitated for four days that she did not even have enough energy to brush her teeth.

At the end of the fourth day she experienced an irregular heartbeat. She was not alarmed since she had a history of irregular heartbeats all her life. They usually lasted two to three minutes and then disappeared.

In the past, her doctor had prescribed Lanoxin, a heart regulating medication. She took it for 13 years, but stopped taking it 10 years ago because the condition did not improve.

This time, the irregular heartbeat started at 5:30 p.m. and continued through the night. In the morning she contacted a cardiologist who said she should be seen immediately. At 11 a.m. the doctor gave her an electrocardiogram and said it was essential to stop the irregular heartbeat (atrial fibrillation) he saw on the EKG immediately. He told her she had to go directly to the hospital.

She got to the emergency room at 2 p.m. Her heart rhythm was monitored and, just as they were about to administer therapeutic heart regulating agents (a beta blocker and a blood thinner), a doctor glanced at the monitor and noticed the patient's heart had returned to a normal rhythm. She was discharged from the hospital.

The doctor prescribed daily doses of Lanoxin and one 325 mg aspirin daily. Jennifer was told to return in two weeks for an echocardiogram and a blood test. When she returned, the electrocardiogram and echocardiogram and blood tests were normal. The latter was to check her thyroid gland because hyperthyroidism can cause an irregular heartbeat. An irregular heartbeat can also be caused by food allergies, low blood sugar, anxiety or a virus infection. No other diagnostic procedures were performed.

She was told to remain on the medication for six months and then return for further evaluation. Three and a half weeks later she became severely constipated and developed hemorrhoids from straining. Since she never had any problems with her bowels, she attributed this to the medication.

She stopped taking the medication and incorporated stool softening foods in her diet, consisting of fruits, vegetables, whole grains and an abundance of water. She also drank four ounces of hot prune juice twice a day, took two ounces of aloe vera gel three times a day and drank a cup of Laci Le Beau tea after her dinner. Even with this regimen, it took three weeks for her bowel function to return to normal. And the hemorrhoids finally disappeared after she used Vitamin E topically following all bowel movements.

This could all have been avoided if the doctor had realized that the atrial fibrillation could have been triggered by the virus. In her case the medication was totally unnecessary and only successful in complicating her life.

Supplements to insure regularity of the heartbeat are:

- Hawthorne berries (an herb)
- Magnesium
- Taurine (amino acid)
- CoEnzyme Q-10
- L-Carnitine

Inappropriate Measures

Following an accident, a seven-year-old female ruptured her spleen. Emergency surgery was performed to remove the spleen due to profuse internal bleeding. Her recovery was uneventful. As a routine procedure following a splenectomy, she was vaccinated against pneumonia and at a follow-up visit, the doctor suggested small doses of penicillin continuously to prevent infection.

The spleen in located in the upper left abdomen behind the ribs. Its function is to destroy worn-out blood cells and remove them from the body. It also aids the immune system, helps produce antibodies against bacteria and viruses and manufactures lymphocytes.

Two months later the child started to complain of itching in the anal area. Her mother noticed a red ring around the child's anus. She also had abdominal bloating, cracks between her toes and cognitive impairment and fatigue. These were the side effects of the antibiotic which depleted the friendly bacteria in the gut needed for digestion and absorption of food.

The doctor said these symptoms would disappear without treatment, that they were a phase of the body's ability to adjust to the antibiotic. However the symptoms worsened.

A holistic doctor who was seen for a second opinion recognized the symptoms of a yeast infection. She recommended high doses of acidophilus bifidus to replace the friendly bacteria. After a few weeks, the yeast infection disappeared. There are times when antibiotic therapy *is* necessary, but appropriate measures to counter the side effects should always be incorporated.

Back Surgery Backfires

After many years of abusing his back, James, a piano mover, developed such severe pain that he was forced to stop working. His primary care physician examined him and said the condition was due to muscle strain. Muscle relaxants and hot baths were recommended. James diligently took his medicine and soaked in the tub, but after two weeks with no improvement he returned to the doctor.

He was referred to an orthopedic surgeon who recommended an MRI which showed herniated discs in the fourth and fifth lumbar area. The surgeon said that was the cause of the problem and suggested a laminectomy (a surgical procedure which fuses the vertebrae).

Fifty percent of all back operations fail and cause increased pain and immobility. A study was performed on 50 individuals with no symptoms of back problems. The MRI diagnosed the majority of these individuals with herniated discs and slight stenosis of the spinal column. The conclusion of the study was that, in most cases, the dysfunctional part of the spine does not necessarily cause pain.

This information, however, was not relayed to the patient. But when the surgical procedure was performed and there was *no* improvement, only more agony, James found this out for himself.

A co-worker of James's with a similar problem sought a nonsurgical approach instead. He consulted a chiropractor who performed the appropriate spinal adjustments, recommended massage therapy and a regimen of back exercises. The chiropractor referred him to a holistic practitioner who suggested weight loss, anti-inflammatory supplements and relaxation techniques. In four weeks he was mobile, most of his pain was eliminated and he was able to return to work.

Another example where staying out of the hospital was better.

Didn't Know Right From Left

When a Tampa, Florida man went into surgery to have his right leg amputated from the knee down, he joked with the attendants to make sure not to remove the wrong leg by mistake.

The man emerged from a fog of anesthesia horrified to discover that, indeed, the *left* leg, which was in perfectly good condition, had been removed from the knee down. The patient's lawyer argued there was absolutely no reason for the mix-up because the right leg which was supposed to have been amputated was covered with sores and gangrenous tissue as a result of deterioration from poor circulation, a condition common to diabetics.

Later, the man's diseased right lower leg was finally amputated at a different hospital, leaving him totally legless and devastated. Though he received a settlement from both the physician and the hospital, the doctor was allowed to keep working. This same doctor was suspended from practice 5 months later, *only* after he amputated the toe of another patient, without her consent.

With horror stories like these, isn't it a good idea to do everything possible to stay out of the hospital?

Almost Worried To Death

When given negative information regarding their physical condition, the psychological effect on a person in tip top condition can be catastrophic enough to initiate a true sickness.

A 35-year-old strong, healthy aerobics instructor, full of vitality, went in for a routine physical and was terrified when her doctor said her electrocardiogram showed evidence of a silent heart attack some time in the past. She was informed that further diagnostic procedures were necessary.

Even though she knew she was in excellent shape and had no symptoms, she was so terrified, she couldn't eat, sleep or concentrate. And this affected her professional and private life to such an extent that her relationship with her boyfriend became strained, and people began dropping out of her aerobics classes.

The dreaded follow-up tests included a thallium stress and an angiogram. Both were negative, proving that the original diagnosis was wrong, but the damage had already been done because the patient had had to endure the anxiety and fear of a future disabling heart attack which never would have occurred.

Physicians should never tell any of their patients that they are in desperate circumstances until, and if, absolute proof of this is evident from further diagnostic procedures. All too often a false positive result can be misconstrued as a serious illness, and telling the patient this result can have a cataclysmic effect on them.

Nosed Out

A popular sinus decongestant spray has been shown to cause such disastrous effects that its use has been questioned and it may possibly be banned.

A worker in a burlap bag factory had chronic sinusitis diagnosed as an allergic reaction to the dust and the material involved in the manufacture of the burlap. An allergist recommended medication, and an ear, nose and throat specialist recommended surgery. The man did not wish to have surgery and opted for the allergist's recommendations, but the medication had side effects of sleepiness and dryness so he decided to stop taking it and try an over-the-counter decongestant spray.

He was delighted when his condition improved almost 100 percent after three days of using the spray. He continued using it and, thinking the condition was cured, stopped it after two weeks.

Within three days, the original problem returned. He started using the spray again, but this time the recovery period took a week. Thinking he had stopped too soon the first time, he continued using the spray for a month, then felt well and discontinued its use.

In just one day, the symptoms returned so he started using the spray again. But, he began to notice a burning sensation in his nasal passages with each application so he stopped using it again, and again his symptoms returned, this time with a vengeance.

He went back to the ear, nose and throat specialist who told him he had burned out the endothelial membrane lining his nasal passages by his prolonged use of this decongestant. A procedure was performed to repair the membrane and three medications were prescribed to prevent the recurrence of the condition. He was told he had to take these medications for the rest of his life in order to keep the lining of his nasal passages intact. His original problem of allergy-induced sinusitis was not addressed.

The medications he was forced to take caused numerous side effects, including weight gain, constipation, hair loss, stomach pain and a severe worsening of the sinusitis.

All of this—the surgery, the hospitalization, the medications—could have been avoided if the original problem with his sinuses had been treated simply by wearing a filter-type face mask at work, and by using natural, helpful antihistamines such as drinking three quarts of water daily and taking high amounts of bioflavanoids, Vitamin C and Vitamin B^6.

Don't Get Stoned

When Howard C. awoke in the middle of the night with intolerable pain in the lower right side of his back, he couldn't fathom what was happening to him. He had never experienced such agony, and when the pain became even more severe, he called the emergency ambulance service.

He was taken to the emergency room where the doctors questioned him about any activity that may have led to the onset of the pain. Nothing could be established by his history, but since he had some burning upon urination, the doctors surmised something was askew in his urinary tract.

An intravanous pyelogram (X-ray of the kidney, ureters and bladder) was ordered and showed a one centimeter calcium oxalate stone lodged at the junction of the kidney and ureter. This prevented the transit of urine from the kidney through the ureter and the resulting build-up of urine caused excessive pressure on the kidney and led to the severe pain.

Conservative therapy was recommended for a one week period. This included medication for pain and drinking large enough amounts of water to make the urine run clear. After being on this treatment for a week with no relief, another pyelogram was taken. This one showed that the stone had migrated from the kidney area to the lower end of the ureter close to the bladder.

Since the stone had moved, another week of conservative therapy was recommended. At times the pain was so severe that Howard actually burst into tears. Note: This pain is on a par with labor pains.

A third pyelogram taken at the end of this week showed the stone had moved into the bladder. Since the ureter was no longer blocked, most of the pain had disappeared except for a slight feeling of pressure upon urination. The urologist said he would most likely pass the stone in a few days.

Howard continued to drink large amounts of water and, to his amazement, upon urinating, a one centimeter (approximately three-eighths inch) diameter stone passed through his penis and dropped into the toilet bowel, relieving him of his horrible pain. He retrieved the stone since the urologist had told him to save it for a chemical analysis.

Analysis showed the stone was formed of calcium oxalate. The doctor said that calcium was binding together in the kidney, causing the formation of the stone. He was told his system was high in calcium and he should therefore refrain from ingesting calcium-rich foods. He was given a list of what foods to avoid and, because he never wanted a repeat of the pain, he diligently adhered to the recommended dietary restrictions.

After a four month period, Howard started to experience pains in his legs, lower back and arms. X-rays of these areas showed stress fractures of his bones, caused by deficiencies in calcium. A dual photon bone density test further showed evidence of early osteoporosis.

By this time Howard was disgusted and started to investigate other avenues of therapy. After reading my first book, ***How To Stay Out Of The Doctor's Office,*** he contacted me.

I ordered specific blood tests which showed the calcium stone build-up was not entirely caused by a high dietary intake of calcium. The significant information my tests revealed was a severe magnesium deficiency. This was not picked up by the urologist's tests which measured the magnesium level only in the serum and not in the blood cell.

Live cell analysis revealed low magnesium levels in the cell which allow calcium to inundate the cell and cause the formation of a stone. Most kidney stones are the calcium oxalate type and can usually be passed by consuming large amounts of water.

If they do not pass, they can usually be retrieved through a cystoscope. In this procedure, a lighted tube is inserted into the bladder and forceps grab the stone. If cystoscopy is not successful, a new procedure called lithotripsy utilizes ultrasound rays to blast the stone into tiny particles that can be flushed out naturally.

In Howard's case, my recommendation was 500 mg of magnesium three times daily to balance his calcium ratio, and Vitamin B^6, 100 mg three times daily for a diuretic effect. I also instructed him to drink at least eight to ten glasses of water every day until at least one urination a day was clear in color.

He followed my recommendations and also started consuming calcium-rich foods again to bring his bone density levels back to normal. Soon he was on his way back to his previous good health. The pain in his back and arms disappeared, and he has had no further problems with kidney stones.

The Cantor Sings No More

A 70-year-old cantor, long praised for singing the prayers at the synagogue, went for his annual checkup, generally confident about his health. The doctor questioned him about his general health and physical activities. The cantor said he felt well and healthy, played 18 holes of golf three times a week and also participated in doubles tennis.

Periodically, he said, while playing tennis he experienced an occasional, slight angina which disappeared upon resting. Otherwise he could perform all other activities plus his occupational responsibilities.

A physical examination consisting of blood pressure readings, blood tests and an electrocardiogram revealed no abnormalities. The cantor was relieved to learn that all the tests were negative. However, his joy was short-lived when the doctor stated that, "to play it safe" at his age, he should have an angiogram.

Since all tests were negative, he questioned the doctor who was insistent that he have the angiogram performed. If not, the doctor said, he would not be responsible if the patient had a full-blown heart attack. The cantor was so intimidated that he acquiesced.

The angiogram revealed an 82 percent blockage in the main coronary artery and a 92 percent blockage in the descending artery. Immediate bypass surgery was recommended, despite statistical studies that have shown that, with very slight angina symptoms such as this man experienced, there is only a one to two percent chance of death. This information was not imparted to the patient.

The bypass surgery was performed and, during the procedure, nerves leading to the vocal cords were severed which caused the cantor to lose his voice and therefore his job in the synagogue. Worse, after recovering from surgery and resuming his athletic activities, he continued to experience the same slight angina. This shows the futility and the potential for bad side effects of this overperformed surgical procedure that in most cases is not needed.

This man's heart disease could have been reversed by a nutritional program comprised of specific heart supplements, a vegetarian diet, an exercise regimen, stress reduction and chelation therapy. But of course this method does not reap the financial rewards of surgery, and patients who opt for the nutritional approach are looked upon by their peers as oddballs and eccentrics.

Chemotherapy Strikes Out Again

A noted medical journalist, who wrote for a large city newspaper, contracted breast cancer. Knowledgeable about the ins and outs and misuses of orthodox treatment for the disease, she still went along with conventional recommendations for a mastectomy and chemotherapy.

She appeared to recover and continued with her professional life and the raising of her children. All went well for a few years until, at an annual checkup, she heard the dreaded news that the cancer had spread to her lung.

She returned to the hospital where she had been treated originally. A bone marrow transplant was recommended at this hospital that had performed the original mastectomy. Although dismayed by the cold, seemingly uncaring attitude of the doctors she talked with, and although she investigated other hospitals where the staff seemed more compassionate, the original hospital's closeness to her home and the support of her family made her disregard her negative gut feelings and opt to have the bone marrow transplant done there.

During the course of her therapy, the staff mistakenly administered four times the required amount of chemotherapy to her, causing violent illness, swelling of her body from retained fluid, protruding eyes and intense vomiting. She even regurgitated the lining of her intestinal wall.

Safeguards regarding chemotherapy administration were not followed in this case and the wrong dosage was administered every day until, by the third day, she had regurgitated the entire lining of her gut. When her frantic husband questioned the doctors, they said it was a normal reaction to a bone marrow transplant. In addition, although her electrocardiograms were abnormal, they were completely overlooked by the staff. Cytoxan, the chemotherapy used on her, is known to damage the heart.

After the patient died, an autopsy showed no visible signs of breast cancer so they won the battle but lost the war.

Chemotherapy acts by destroying rapidly dividing cancer cells. However, it also destroys all other rapidly dividing cells in the body. Bone marrow cells divide rapidly and are needed to fight infection, but these were also destroyed by the high chemotherapy dosage.

This type of therapy continues despite countless cases similar to the above. Patients are kept in the dark and never given the true statistics regarding success and failure rates of chemotherapy and surgery. Instead, they are given a response rate, interpreted by the unknowledgeable as a cure, but which, in actuality, usually lasts for an average of 28 days.

The public is so brainwashed through fear and intimidation that even a knowledgeable, respected medical writer fell prey and suffered fatal consequences.

Four Day Diabetes Cure

Harvey C., a museum curator and an adult-onset diabetic, came to me because he was worried about his weight, his insomnia and the high amount of insulin his doctor prescribed for him. He was injecting himself with 130 units daily. This is considered a very high amount for Type II diabetes.

I asked if his insulin levels had been taken and he wanted to know why they were necessary. I explained that, with adult-onset diabetes, most of the problem is not due to lack of insulin. Diabetes is the inability to process glucose which is derived only from carbohydrates.

Due to his doctor's inability to consider symptoms and his reliance on the blood sugar readings only, it's likely he was overprescribing insulin, as is often the case. Most likely the pancreas is overproducing insulin, but the body is insensitive to it so the high blood sugar readings won't go lower.

This condition can be completely rectified by simply eliminating the need for the pancreas to produce so much insulin. Harvey didn't know what carbohydrates were so I explained the difference between carbohydrate-type food, which is any food grown in the field, and fat and protein which are derived from fish, poultry, meat and dairy products, and told him to stay away from carbohydrates.

Harvey then exclaimed, "You mean it's that simple!" I said it was and explained that synthetic insulin injected into the body is atherogenic and causes the destruction of the internal lining of the arteries, causing leakage and plaque accumulation and leading to heart disease.

I recommended a high protein, low carbohydrate diet and the addition of specific supplements to aid his glucose metabolism. Supplements included chromium picolinate, zinc, magnesium, biotin and vanadyl sulfate, all available in health food stores.

Within four days his blood sugar reverted to near-normal levels. As an additional bonus to being on this diet, he also lost weight and his insomnia disappeared.

Dietitian Sees The Light

A dietitian in a major teaching hospital was diagnosed with colitis. Conventional treatment consisted of medication to depress the sympathetic nervous system and stimulate the parasympathetic nervous system. One cause of colitis is presumed to be a malfunction of the sympathetic nervous system which promotes the production of adrenalin, causing hyperactivity of the colon and leading to constant diarrhea and inflammation. An underactive parasympathetic nervous system can cause constipation.

She took the medication over a five year period, whenever her symptoms appeared. The condition progressively worsened, but its underlying cause was never investigated and the medications offered only palliative relief.

As an orthodox dietitian, holistic therapy was the furthest thing from her mind. At her colitis support group, several participants related that they were having excellent results following the treatments recommended by a holistic doctor. She inquired about these treatments and was told that they included investigating and treating underlying yeast problems, food allergies and parasites, and determining if a hyperactive thyroid was causing too rapid a transit time.

The dietitian asked her gastroenterologist about these tests and he said they were meaningless and that she should continue with his program. Since she was not improving, she asked a member of the support group to recommend a practitioner and was referred to me. I recommended a gluten-free and a sugarless, yeast-free diet, with added aloe vera gel and high amounts of acidophilus to rebuild her intestinal flora. I also gave her a supplement to destroy parasites and told her to take digestive enzymes with her meals. They facilitate digestion by helping to eliminate microscopic particles of food that don't get digested and cause food allergies. Within three weeks, most of her symptoms were gone and she was overwhelmed by the success of the treatment.

Gynecologist Strikes Out

At her annual, routine gynecological checkup, Lucille M., a 33-year-old married woman hoping to have a child, was told she had polycystic disease of the ovaries. Polycystic disease is a malfunction of the ovary whereby, instead of producing a viable egg, a fluid-filled cyst is formed.

Although Lucille had none of the usual symptoms, such as spotting, pain, pressure on the bladder and rectum, and fever, the doctor recommended a total hysterectomy. Lucille and her husband were devastated since they both wanted a family. They inquired about alternatives to a hysterectomy and were told there were none, and that, in fact, without a total hysterectomy in the near future, she would be at risk for dire consequences.

She went for a second opinion and this doctor concurred with the original doctor's advice, saying it was futile for her to continue to seek an opinion against surgery.

Lucille was referred to me by a friend and, after consulting with her, I recommended she have blood tests done to ascertain female hormone levels. Neither gynecologist had recommended these tests, or any tests to determine whether the estrogen and progesterone receptor sites on the ovaries were implicated.

The test results showed her progesterone levels were extremely low and were causing an overactivity of estrogen, a possible cause of the cysts. Armed with this information, I instituted a simple program consisting of topical application of Progest Cream, a product containing extract of wild yams. After three months of this natural therapy, a gynecologist found no evidence of cysts. Two months after that, to the amazement of her doctor, Lucille became pregnant and the only hospital in her life was for the happy event of the birth of her child, not the unnecessary hysterectomy.

Dire Consequences Of Unnecessary Testing

Ellen R,. a graphic artist, was told by her doctor that it was essential for everyone over 50 to undergo a lower GI to rule out colon cancer, which he referred to as a silent killer. Since she was completely symptom-free, she balked at having the procedure, but when the doctor said it was as important as a mammogram, she acquiesced.

Preparation for the examination consisted of fasting and bowel-cleansing with liquid magnesium citrate the evening before the test was to be performed. Ellen was up all night going to the bathroom and eventually experienced anal discomfort from all the bowel movements. The following morning she was made even more uncomfortable because she was instructed to use a laxative-type suppository.

A lower GI is a barium enema done under a fluoroscopic machine. The test was also uncomfortable and proved negative. However, for the week following the test, she was severely constipated because some of the barium had solidified and was clogging the crevices of the colon.

Ellen subsequently developed severe hemorrhoids from all the straining, and a hemorrhoidectomy was recommended. Following the surgery, packing was inserted in her anus. Two nurses gave her large doses of stool softener. The amount was excessive and caused bloating and so much downward pressure that it displaced the packing and caused hemorrhaging.

She was rushed back to the operating room to control the bleeding. Since emergency blood transfusions were necessary, she now lives in fear for her life worrying about the possibility of having been given HIV-infected blood that could lead to AIDS. This patient's original problem *wasn't* one, yet now she does have a problem.

This above scenario is all too typical of unnecessary testing with complete disregard for the patient's well-being. In the majority of cases, for any testing procedure performed on asymptomatic individuals, the general percentage of positive results is less than two percent. This means that 98 percent of people tested have no disease. Yet all the tests are forced upon them by fear and intimidation.

Twice As Likely To Die In America

Two hours into the medical treatment that was cleansing Sue's blood, she screamed, pulled at her hair and vomited, reported *The New York Times.*

Panic spread at the New Mexico hospital as five other people undergoing the same kidney dialysis treatment also screamed in intense, unexpected pain. Even though the nurses immediately turned off the machines, and even though most of the patients recovered, *Sue died within six hours.*

This tragic episode was attributed to human error. A technician had mistakenly thrown a switch to rinse the dialysis machines while the patients were hooked up to them. This rinse, rather than the correct blood-cleansing solution, had been shot into their bloodstreams, causing their cells to break down.

Some experts, however, said the machines were old and outdated—with no alarm-warning systems. The fact is, an American dialysis patient is *twice* as likely to die as a dialysis patient in Western Europe or Japan.

58 Conclusion

This book is about *not* going to the hospital, but in the event it does become necessary and you are unable to avoid hospitalization, the following information will help you protect yourself. Don't be afraid to speak up. You may upset some of the staff but you will save yourself a great deal of unnecessary anguish.

1. If you are having elective surgery performed, talk to your doctor about banking your blood beforehand. There is still serious concern over the risks involved in transfusions, and should you need blood, your are safer using your own.

2. Before any surgical procedure, remind the entire staff what is to be done. If possible, talk to the head operating room nurse before the surgery.

3. Refuse to have a urinary catheter inserted into your bladder for the convenience of the hospital staff. The catheter is a vehicle for the transmission of bacteria into your urinary tract. Before you are admitted, ask your doctor if it is a medical necessity for your condition. If it is unavoidable, have the nurses check its drainage on a regular basis.

On the subject of nurses, there is an alarming trend towards cutting costs by replacing registered nurses (RN's) with the less schooled, less skilled licensed practical nurses (LPN's) or just plain nurse's assistants (NA's). You have a right to know whether or not the nurse attending you is a fully qualified registered nurse. If not, ask for one who is. You can look at the name badge, if they are wearing one, to see what initials follow the name.

4. Request a list of all medications to be administered and the exact dosage. Note the color, size and shape of each pill so

you will be able to see if a mistake has been made. Keep the list by your bedside and refer to it whenever medication is administered. If something seems different, question the nurse before taking it.

5. If you are in a semi-private room, be sure the other person does not have a severe mental problem or infectious disease. If you suspect either, insist upon changing your room.

6. As soon as you are in your room, inform the nurse that you are going to test your call button to be sure it works. Ask what a reasonable response time is. If you have to use the call button and do not get attention in a reasonable period of time, use your telephone. You can call the hospital and ask to be connected to the nursing station in your area, the patient relations department, the administrator or your doctor.

7. Ask to see the results of your laboratory reports and try to get copies of them for documentation that may be necessary at a later date. You have the right to this information.

8. Insist that enough blood be drawn at one time for all laboratory studies. All too often technicians from different departments do not communicate with each other and subject patients to repeated venipunctures. There is no reason why they can't all use blood from one vial.

9. Request a consultation with the dietitian and inform him or her about any food allergies you may have. Be sure to avoid all sugary-type foods and foods high in fat content. Eat lots of fruits and vegetables since they are high in oxygen content which is needed for tissue repair.

10. Before anyone touches you for any reason whatsoever, even to take your blood pressure, be sure they wash their hands. Hospital staff often wear rubber gloves. This is an OSHA (Occupational Safety Hazards Act) regulation for the protection of the staff, not for you. Ask them to put on fresh gloves in your presence.

Visitors should also wash their hands. It is absolutely essential that anyone who touches you or any of your things wash their hands since many infections are spread through hand contact. Anyone who leaves your room, even for a brief period, must wash their hands upon returning. If the housekeeping staff balks at your request, remind them that you also insist that physicians and administrators wash their hands.

11. Ask your surgeon to put it in writing that he or she will be the one performing the surgery. All too often well-known surgeons only do part of the surgery and allow residents to do the rest. Ask about the surgeon's complication rate and infection rate.

12. Discuss with your doctor in advance exactly what tests will be ordered. Inquire whether any of them are painful or dangerous and if the tests' advantages outweigh their risks. If they could lead to complications more serious than your condition, ask what will happen if you don't have them done. Hazardous tests involving radiation or nuclear medicine should be kept to a minimum.

13. Call your department of health and inquire about the infection rate of the hospital.

14. The anesthesiologist is every bit as important as the surgeon. More than keeping you asleep, it is their job to keep you alive. Talk to the anesthesiologist before the day of surgery, make sure he or she is board certified, and get it in writing that he or she will be in the operating room with you. If you get double talk about checking in or if you don't feel confident with that person, ask your surgeon to find you a different anesthesiologist, and make sure you meet him or her ahead of time.

This is particularly important now because the HMO-driven hospital rules are causing patients to have less and less pre- and post-operative contact with their anesthesiologists. This is considered something of a scandal by those involved in hospital care.

15. Meet the patient's representative, who might also be known as the patient's advocate or ombudsman, as soon as possible after you are admitted. Find out his or her name, phone number and available hours. If a problem arises, this person acts as an intermediary between you and the doctors and department heads and administrators.

16. Prior to admission, tell your doctor you plan to continue taking your vitamin and mineral supplements and will bring your own with you. Institutional food may not supply the nutrients

you need for your recovery. Make sure to get his confirmation of this in writing.

17. Find out the last time before surgery that you are allowed to eat. If any food is brought to you after that time, don't eat it, since serious complications could arise if food is in your stomach when anesthesia is administered.

Know Your Rights

Above all, know your rights. Hospitals accredited by the Joint Commission of Accredited Health Care Organizations are required to prominently display a *Patient's Bill of Rights.* A copy should be handed to you upon admission. If it's not, request a copy.

The wording of the *Patient's Bill of Rights* may vary from hospital to hospital, but should always include the following:

1. You have the right to considerate and respectful care.
2. You have the right to be well-informed about your condition, possible treatments and likely outcome in language you can understand.
3. You have the right to know by name all people treating you.
4. You have the right to consent to, or refuse a particular treatment. If you do refuse a recommended treatment, you will still receive necessary care.
5. You have the right to a living will or health care proxy. These are documents that express your choice regarding future care. If you have these documents, be sure your family, your doctor and the hospital receive copies.
6. You have the right to privacy.
7. You have the right to confidentiality. All records pertaining to your care are confidential unless you give permission to release them. If the records are released to your insurance company, the hospital should emphasize that the records are confidential.
8. You have the right to review your records and have the information explained to you.
9. You have the right to know if the hospital has relationships with educational institutions, insurers or other health care providers that could influence your treatment and care.

10. You have the right to expect that the hospital will give you necessary services to the best of its ability. If transferring you to another hospital is recommended, you will be informed of all risks, benefits and alternatives, and you will not be transferred unless and until the other institution has agreed to accept you.

11. You have the right to consent or refuse to take part in research or experimentation affecting your care. Should you decline to participate, you will still receive the most effective care the hospital otherwise provides.

12. You have the right to be informed about realistic care alternatives if hospital care is no longer necessary or appropriate.

13. You have the right to know about hospital rules and regulations that apply to your conduct and well-being.

14. You have the right to know about charges and payments and the right to have your bill explained in detail regardless of the payment method.

15. You have the right to know about and to contact resources such as patient representatives and ethics committees whose function is to assist you in resolving problems and answering questions.

16. You have the right to be free from mental and physical abuse and free from chemical and physical restraints unless authorized in writing by a physician for a specified and limited period of time.

17. You have the right to refuse to be examined by medical students, interns and residents.

Be Well-Informed

By being well-informed, participating in decisions regarding your treatment and communicating openly with health care professionals, your hospital stay should improve your health, not destroy it.

About The Authors

Dr. Edward M. Wagner and Sylvia Goldfarb are co-authors of the bestseller, ***How To Stay Out Of The Doctor's Office, An Encyclopedia For Alternative Healing***, published by Instant Improvement, Inc.

Dr. Wagner has been a practicing nutritional medical counselor in the Philadelphia area for the past thirteen years. He has appeared on numerous radio and television programs and now has his own popular radio program in the Philadelphia area.

He is the former Assistant Director of the Pennsylvania branch of the American Nutritional Medical Association. He has a Diploma in Nutrition from the Nutritionist's Institute of America, a Certificate from Dr. Jenks School of Herbalism and Iridology and a Certificate from Wild Rose College of Natural Healing (Vitamins and Minerals).

Sylvia Goldfarb is a writer specializing in medical topics. Some publications her articles have appeared in include, *Today's OR Nurse, Focus, Fodor's Guidebooks, Veggie Times, Natural Body and Fitness, Delaware Valley Magazine and Today's Secretary.*

She serves as a faculty member and judge of the Philadelphia Writer's Conference and gives writing seminars on cruise ships.

Sylvia is a graduate of Skidmore College and a member of the Author's Guild.

Index

G

H

I

J

K

L

M

Q

R

S

T

U

V

W

X

Y

Z